The Conquest of Pain

The Conquest of Pain

Peter Fairley

MICHAEL JOSEPH

LONDON

To Charles, who succeeded

First published in Great Britain by
Michael Joseph Limited
52 Bedford Square
London WC1B 3EF
1978

© 1978 by Peter Fairley

ISBN 0 7181 1646 1

Filmset by D P Media Limited,
Hitchin, Herts
Printed and bound in Great Britain by
Billing & Sons Limited, Guildford, Surrey

Contents

AUTHOR'S FOREWORD

This book has been written for layman and specialist alike – normally, incompatible audiences. To assist the layman, all technical discussion in detail has been printed in smaller type, so that he or she may move more rapidly through the book on stepping stones of simplicity.

PETER FAIRLEY

Introduction

ACCIDENT AT CHIPPING NORTON

The bowler was 6ft 3in. tall, lithe in action, and Australian. I really did not fancy opening the batting to him at all – not on an iron-hard wicket – but there was little I could do about it as he pounded up to the stumps. . . . Sure enough, his first ball ricocheted off a length and smashed into my left hand as it gripped the handle. The pain was excruciating. I flung aside the bat, flicked my hand vigorously, pumped up and down a few times; and gave up. P. Fairley . , . retired hurt . . . 0.

All the groundsman had was a bottle of aspirin tablets. I swallowed two and took myself off to hospital. Waiting for an X-ray in the Fracture Clinic, I started to think about pain. Why did my hand hurt so much? Could bones feel pain? Was it true that the only part of the body insensitive to pain is the outer layer of the brain itself? And if so, why?

I also thought about aspirin. A powerful drug indeed; just two little tablets had considerably dulled the pain in my hand. Yet you could buy it freely over the counter in a chemist's shop. How did it work? Who discovered it?

Back home, nursing a fractured finger, I looked up 'Aspirin' in the dictionary: 'A sedative drug composed of acetylsalicylic acid'. I looked up 'Acetyl': 'the basis of the acetic series'. I looked up 'Acetic': 'of the nature of, or pertaining to, vinegar'. *Vinegar*? Under 'Salicyl' I found this: 'the diatomic radical of salicylic acid – from Latin, *salix*, a willow'. *Willow*?

Vinegar and willow. Could they really be the basis for aspirin? Next morning I rang Eric Engler, Information Services Manager at Reckitt & Colman, the Hull-based company which I knew made aspirin. 'How was aspirin first discovered?' I asked him. Eric explained that the first scientific reference to the pain and fever-reducing properties of salicylic acid – the basic active ingredient of aspirin, and contained in the leaves of the willow tree – was in a paper presented to the Royal Society in London in 1763, by a gentleman calling himself 'the Reverend Edmund Stone' at the top of the paper but signing himself 'Edward Stone' at the bottom. He had come from Chipping Norton.

A *clergyman* involved with vinegar, willow trees and the practice of medicine? Eric explained that the vinegar bit came later, but offered to send me a photocopy of Stone's paper to the Royal Society. This is how it began:

> XXXII. *An Account of the succefs of the Bark of the Willow in the Cure of Agues. In a Letter to the Right Honourable George Earl of Macclesfield, Prefident of R. S. from the Rev. Mr.* Edmund Stone, *of* Chipping-Norton *in* Oxfordfhire.
>
> My Lord,
>
> Read June 2d, 1763. **A**Mong the many ufeful difcoveries, which this age hath made, there are very few which, better deferve the attention of the public than what I am going to lay before your Lordfhip.
>
> There is a bark of an Englifh tree, which I have found by experience to be a powerful aftringent, and very efficacious in curing aguifh and intermitting diforders.
>
> About fix years ago, I accidentally tafted it, and was furprifed at its extraordinary bitternefs; which immediately raifed me a fufpicion of its having the properties of the Peruvian bark. As this tree delights in a moift or wet foil, where agues chiefly abound, the general maxim, that many natural maladies carry their cures along with them, or that their remedies lie not far from their caufes, was fo very appofite to this particular cafe, that I could not help applying it. . . .

And this is how it ended:

> . . . cinnamon or lateritious colour, which I believe is the cafe with the Peruvian bark and powders.
>
> I have no other motives for publifhing this valuable fpecific, than that it may have a fair and full trial in all its variety of circumftances and fituations, and that the world may reap the benefits accruing from it. For thefe purpofes I have given this long and minute account of it,

and which I would not have troubled your Lordſhip with, was I not fully perſuaded of the wonderful efficacy of this Cortex Salignus in agues and intermitting caſes, and did I not think, that this perſuaſion was ſufficiently ſupported by the manifold experience, which I have had of it.

I am, my Lord,

with the profoundeſt ſubmiſſion and reſpect,

Chipping-Norton,   your Lordſhip's moſt obedient
Oxfordshire,
April 25, 1763.   humble Servant

Edward Stone.

By the time I had read the whole discourse my curiosity was thoroughly aroused. What was a clergyman doing wandering around wet ground in Chipping Norton, concerned about 'aguish' – a word commonly used for malarial fever – and taking samples of willow bark? And who were the fifty souls to whom he had administered his home-made salicylate? There, at the point of origin of the world's most widely used drug, was a 200-year-old mystery which nobody had attempted to solve. I set off for Chipping Norton.

Chipping Norton – 'Chippie' to locals – is an Oxfordshire market town which clings, somewhat uncomfortably, to the side of a hill. In the valley at the bottom a brook meanders through reeds and nettlebeds, from one end of the town to the other. The brook is subject to flooding, and in fact the flat ground to either side of it was once marshland.

I parked my car by the churchyard, walked down an overgrown footpath, and began to pick my way through cow-pats and hoof-marks to where a line of woods began. I walked a quarter of a mile before I found a willow tree, but it was a magnificent specimen – huge, and clearly very old. Was this the tree which Edward (or was it Edmund?) Stone had 'accidentally tasted'? I removed a strip of bark and went in search of the vicar.

No, he didn't know who the Reverend Edward Stone was. Nor Edmund. No, so far as he knew, neither was buried in his churchyard. But why didn't I speak to David Eddershaw?

David Eddershaw is schools organizer at the Oxford City and County Museum at Woodstock, a historian and an authority on 'Chippie'. 'Funny you should be interested,' he said, 'we had an American over here a couple of years ago, trying to find out who Edward Stone was. Couldn't help him much at the time, but since then we've discovered a little.'

Mr Eddershaw explained that records kept in the vaults of a local bank contained minutes of a meeting of the bailiffs and burgesses of Chipping Norton in 1725, at which a sum of money had been voted for the planting of fifty sallow (willow) trees on common land adjoining the brook. He offered to search for the Enclosure Award of 1770 on which all the names of landowners in Chipping Norton at the time would be entered, together with a map of their titles.

To our great delight, the Award showed a hump-shaped patch of about twenty-two acres bordering the brook and abutting common land, and clearly assigned to 'The Revd. Edward Stone'. I could hardly wait to take a copy of the map back to Chipping Norton and explore. I drove to the west end of the town, out into farmland and parked at the kennels of the Heythrop Hunt. Taking a footpath down to the brook, I was excited to see that it was lined with willow trees.

Brooks normally change course very little. It was possible to work out from the wiggles on the map and the twists of its banks in real life, exactly where the Reverend Edward Stone's land had begun and ended. And there – running along the water's edge, on what must certainly have been marshy ground in previous centuries – stood fifteen fine old willow trees. One of them, by a five-bar gate, had virtually split in two.

The birthplace of aspirin! But who was Edward Stone?

Answering that took longer. My impression that he was seeking a remedy for malaria had been fostered by an article on aspirin by H. O. J. Collier, published in *Scientific American* in 1963. This had reproduced part of Stone's letter to the President of the Royal Society, with its reference to 'aguish' and 'intermittent disorders', and had added the comment 'a description of malaria'. It had also stated 'the bark tasted extraordinarily bitter, as does cinchona, the Peruvian bark that was then acknowledged to be the sovereign remedy for malaria'.

What was the connection between an English clergyman and malaria, a disease quite uncommon in Britain at that time?

I thought, at first, that he might have been attached to a military unit as chaplain and contracted the disease while the unit was on foreign service. I visualized a crimped-up old man dressed in black, with bones like a skeleton, a man pale and shivering as the fever gripped him from time to time, long after his discharge. But military historians assured me that it was not the Army's practice in those days to send chaplains overseas.

I thought he might have been a missionary and been bitten by the parasite mosquito in some jungle swamp; but if he had, then neither history nor the Church had recorded it. Neither Crockford's Clerical List, nor the Clergy List, nor the Ecclesiastical Directory, nor the Clerical Guide, nor any of the medical registers went back that far. Nor did the records at Somerset House.

Confidence returned when a researcher friend, Karen de Groot, discovered in the Oxford County Record Office a set of volumes entitled *The Alumni Oxoniensis*. In the one spanning the period 1715–1886 was the following entry: 'Stone, Edward, s. Edward of Westminster (city), cler. Wadham Coll.; matric. 10 Oct 1758 aged 15 (b.1743); B.A. 1762, M.A. 1767; rector of Horsendon, Bucks 1769; vicar of Stagsdon, Beds; perp. curate Princes Risborough; J.P. Oxon and Bucks; died 15 Feb 1811'.

Another record at the County Office revealed that this Edward Stone was a party in the Deed (Chipping Norton) – a kind of landowners' list – in 1763. I was sure we were back on the right track. But what was a young man of twenty, later to be involved in the ministry at Horsendon, Stagsdon and Princes Risborough, doing with land at Chipping Norton? And why was he wandering through its marshes? And why, when so young, was he writing to the President of the Royal Society? The parish records for Chipping Norton were no help. Nor were those for Cornwell, Salford or Overnorton, which adjoined Edward Stone's land. I drew a blank, too, with tombstones in the area.

Some friends set off for Horsendon, Stagsdon and Princes Risborough. One of them, Rosemary Kent, learned from the County Archivist at Aylesbury that a Reverend Edward Stone, married to a Miss Elizabeth Grubb, had died at Chipping Norton and on 2 December 1768 had been buried in Horsendon churchyard. Was this the father of the young experimenter who had written to the Royal Society? Or was *he* actually the author of the paper? The latter now seemed more likely. Rosemary Kent gives this description of her visit to Horsendon in search of Edward Stone's grave:

Horsendon lies a couple of miles to the south-west of Princes Risborough. The village consists of a few cottages, a large, manor-type house and the church. There are thirty or forty gravestones in the churchyard, most of them twentieth century. A number of broken pieces of gravestone lie scattered about. But apart from providing refuge for wood-lice and spiders, these held no clues.

The church itself is more like a chapel. Services are only held there once a month and the church is kept locked. There are many plaques on its walls and – like much of the stained glass – most of these commemorate different generations of the Grubb family. One John Grubb, who died in 1775, was a Patron of the parish and his remains lie in a vault. But I could find no mention of Edward Stone. I learned, however, that the church was pulled down in 1765 and then rebuilt. Presumably Stone died while the rebuilding was going on, and somehow his grave has been lost.

I was back at square one.

About this time, I had a stroke of luck. Unknown to me, the curriculum for the Nuffield Advanced Course for schools biology studies had landed on the desk of Paul Lister, biology master at Chipping Norton School. In it, on page 426, was the following project:

Edward Stone, a clergyman of Chipping Norton, first described the curative powers of the bark from the willow in 1763. He used extracts of the bark for treating malaria. Incidentally, willow bark tastes very bitter, as does the bark of the Peruvian tree cinchona spp. from which quinine is extracted. In 1829, a substance called 'salicin' was isolated from willow bark, and later salicylic acid was derived from this.
Question: Why is extract of willow bark unlikely to have the same effect as quinine on patients suffering from malaria?

Mr Lister showed it to Ralph Mann, senior history master at the school, who in turn showed it to some of his keenest pupils. 'Who', he asked, 'was the Reverend Edward Stone?' Five fourth-formers – Nicholas Hill, Glenville Fowler, Michael Turner, Colin Seymour and Paul Timms – decided to carry out the investigation as a special project. Letters were dispatched to the Oxford County Records Office and the local parishes which might be able to throw some light on the mystery. The Enclosure Award was examined, the ground inspected. Piece by piece, this picture of the clergyman was built up:

He was fourth in a line of five Edward Stones, two of whom had married women called Elizabeth Grubb (it was not surprising that I had plumped for the wrong generation at first). He was born in Princes Risborough in 1702, the son of a yeoman, and he went to Wadham College, Oxford. After graduating in 1724, he was elected a scholar of the college. Four years later he was ordained 'deacon' by the Bishop of Lincoln and became curate of Saunderton in Buckinghamshire. Shortly afterwards, he was ordained 'priest' by the Bishop of Oxford, and switched to becoming curate at Charlton-on-Otmoor. But he retained his ties with Oxford.

In 1730, his college elected him to a Fellowship and he began lecturing undergraduates in the Humanities. Stone was a voracious reader – in fact, a year later he took over the running of the college library. After another year he became Bursar and then, two years later, Dean; but he still continued as Librarian.

During vacations, the youthful Stone would return home to see his family. They lived at Princes Risborough in Buckinghamshire. His father, Edward, had married twice – the second time into a wealthy land-owning family of the area named Grubb. Elizabeth Grubb, the clergyman's stepmother, had a niece – also named Elizabeth. Whether Stone actually fell in love with her or whether the family merely felt it was a suitable match, is unclear. But Stone returned to Oxford in 1740 (he was then thirty-eight) desirous of marriage; in fact, a marriage settlement had been arranged, giving the couple sixty acres of land in the parish of Owlswick and fifty-nine acres at Horsendon in Buckinghamshire.

The problem was that universities did not permit their Fellows to be married. If he wanted to wed, therefore, he had to leave. For two or three years, it seems, Stone led a frustrating existence, unable to make his mind up what to do. He had, by that time, added the parish church of Horsendon – in the heart of Grubb land – to his list of ministries (he was appointed Rector on 10 March 1737). But presumably the stipend it carried was insufficient for his plans, because he still stayed on at the university.

In June 1741, and possibly because the other Fellows may have grown tired of his tale of unrequited love at high table, Wadham College offered him the living of the parish of Southdrop in Gloucestershire, which it then owned. But Stone turned it down. On 5 December 1741 another man was appointed to the post. Stone quit Oxford. He moved to the parish of Drayton, near Banbury, where he was appointed Rector. At last his income matched his desires, and he married Elizabeth, whom he had then been courting for at least two years. (There were thus two Edward Stones living, both married to Elizabeth Grubbs.) History records that on 29 May 1742 the couple baptized a son . . . Edward. There were then *three* Edward Stones.

After sixteen years at Drayton, Stone had some good fortune. He somehow met a nobleman named Sir Jonathan Cope – probably through the latter's family, who lived in the adjacent parish of Hanwell. Sir Jonathan invited the 56-year-old parson to become his family chaplain, to hold services every Sunday at the family seat at Bruern – site of an old Cistercian abbey – and administer Holy Communion to the family and relatives four times a year. Stone accepted.

He did not move to Bruern itself but to Chipping Norton, where he purchased about twenty-two acres of land (where the money came from, the researchers were unable to discover). It was a steeply sloping plot, traversed by a public right-of-way and extending almost from the Worcester road down to Common Brook (*see figure*). Fringing its southern edge was a line of willow trees, then about thirty years old: very important willow trees.

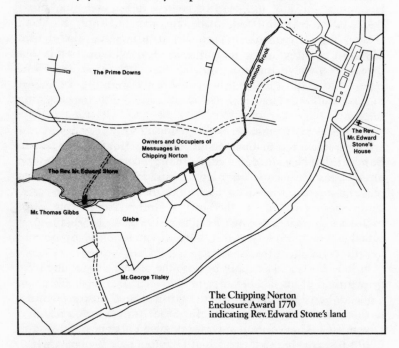

The Chipping Norton
Enclosure Award 1770
indicating Rev. Edward Stone's land

Stone seems to have prospered from the moment he arrived at Chipping Norton. His duties for Sir Jonathan cannot have been arduous, although the eight-mile journey on horseback – along the turnpike as far as Churchill, then over rougher roads to Standbow Bridge and finally to Bruern – cannot have been easy for an elderly clergyman, especially since there was a risk of encountering high-waymen. But he presumably had plenty of time to himself.

His letter to the President of the Royal Society about willow bark was dated 25 April 1763. It was read out at a meeting of the Society on 2 June. During the previous five years, Stone's activities are something of a mystery, although we know he saw his son enter Wadham and take an immediate interest in the Church. In 1761, Stone himself was appointed a Justice of the Peace, a position he held until his death at the age of sixty-six, on 26 November 1768.

Ralph Mann and his fourth-formers had done a magnificent detective job. I now knew who the Reverend Mr Edward Stone was. I knew where his land was. I knew where he was buried. But what was his connection with malaria? And who were the fifty 'patients' to whom he had administered his willow bark concoction? Were they estate workers of Sir Jonathan Cope?

I drove down to Bruern. There is little to it except a few farm-workers' cottages and a magnificient mini-mansion, set in fine grounds, owned by the Hon. Michael Astor. Judy Astor opened the door. 'I'm awfully sorry,' she said when she learned of my mission, 'but the old house burned down around 1780 and the records went with it.'

I drove over to Chipping Norton School. To my great delight, the school was holding an 'open night' for parents, and the five fourth-formers had mounted a special display of their researches. They had also taken samples of willow bark from the banks of Common Brook and pulverized them, as Stone had done. Nicholas Hill explained:

> We went down to one of the willow trees on Stone's old land and stripped off some shoots. We divided them into different growths of one to four years; you can tell by scars on the twigs how long they've been growing. Stone dried his twigs on the outside of a baker's oven for three months, of course, but we couldn't wait that long – we stuck ours in an incubator in the science lab. We wrapped them up in a bit of sacking and baked them at a temperature of about 93°F. for three weeks, and then stripped off the bark. It came off quite easily and we then pulverized it with a pestle and mortar.

Four glass dishes containing a light brown powder were the result, and I sampled each. They were labelled '1st', '2nd', '3rd' and '4th' year, but all tasted equally bitter to me.

'Most people find the fourth-year growth tastes most like aspirin', said Nicholas.

'Have you tried out its fever-reducing properties?' I asked.

'Well,' he answered, 'one woman did come along with a headache and we gave her some. But she went away before we could tell if it had worked!'

The five boys climbed into my car and we drove to Kennel Lane, parked by the kennels of the Heythrop Hunt, walked down the footpath and came to the willow trees. 'Which did you take your twigs from?' I asked. They pointed to the large tree with the split trunk near the five-barred gate. It was just such a tree which I had visualized the Reverend Edward Stone 'accidentally' tasting.

'Any theories as to how he accidentally came to taste the bark?' I asked them.

'Perhaps he tripped, fell against the tree and his teeth sank into it,' suggested Colin Seymour.

The boys also showed me, further up the brook, an old grinding-wheel and some stones – the remnants of a small mill which had stood on the clergyman's land two hundred years previously, and which might (had a bakery been attached) have been the place where he left his twigs to dry for three months before scraping off the bark.

I drove back to London well satisfied. We were still no nearer solving the malaria part of the problem but at least we knew who Stone was and precisely what resulted from his experiment.

Next day, I had another stroke of good fortune. I was passing Culpeper House in Bruton Street, London W1, and suddenly remembered that I had once been supplied with information about the history of herbal medicine, for a TV programme I was doing, by the Society of Herbalists (whose headquarters are at Culpeper House). Unfortunately, I had lost the information.

I went into the delightfully perfumed herb shop on the ground-floor, and came face to face with a book entitled *The Magic of Herbs* (Cape), by David Conway. Chapter 3 was entitled 'The Doctrine of Signatures'.

For the most complete exposition of the Doctrine of Signatures we must turn to a fascinating Neapolitan called Giambattista della Porta. According to him, the places where various plants were wont to grow offered precious information to the perspicacious herbalist. He even asserted that plants common to a particular region would cure the afflictions of its inhabitants, the theory being that the local climate was responsible both for the diseases and their cure.

Della Porta had lived two hundred years before Stone but there was no doubt that, as a Humanist, Stone accepted his medical doctrine; he had even made reference in his letter to the Royal Society to 'the general maxim that many natural maladies carry their cures along with them, or that their remedies lie not far from their causes'.

I read on:

Della Porta's extension of the Doctrine to the actual site favoured by wild plants can be justified by a host of examples. Take the willow tree, for instance, which – because it grows in damp places – was assumed to provide a cure for rheumatism, a condition aggravated, if not caused, by a damp atmosphere.

I read faster:

In accordance with the Doctrine, willow bark was duly prescribed for the easing of rheumatic pain and, curiously, it worked. But still more curious is that when modern science deigned to take an interest in the willow, it discovered a substance to which it gave the name *salicin* (Latin *salix* = willow), once an important stand-by in the treatment of rheumatic fever.

There was the missing link I had been seeking. The Reverend Edward Stone had not necessarily been looking for a cure for malaria but one for rheumatic fever – a common condition in Britain and one from which, quite possibly, he was suffering himself as he approached his fifty-seventh birthday.

I went to the local library and looked up 'ague'. Sure enough, it defined it as 'an acute fever' (1611) and *(fig.)* 'any fit of shaking or shivering'. Malarial fever had been but *one* specialized meaning of the word 'ague' in Edward Stone's day. The word would have been more generally used to describe *any* fever. I still had to surmise how he had found his fifty 'patients ', and my conjectures are described in Chapter 4. But next morning I rang Reckitt & Colman. 'I think I can fill you in a bit about the origins of aspirin,' I told Eric Engler.

This book is the result.

1

What is Pain?

The Greeks had a word for it: 'ponos' (πονος). It meant 'pain'. But what *is* pain?

Pain is many things to many people. It is no respecter of persons and can lay low a millionaire as easily as it can an alley-cat; the only difference is the degree to which the sufferer is able to do something about it. For some sufferers, it can become a way of life. Seeking relief, they hobble and limp from doctor to doctor. Back pain alone, in the Western world, accounts for something like 50 million doctor visits a year; migraine perhaps for 25 million. In America, the cost of surgery to relieve pain – and the cost of analgesic drugs – is estimated to exceed ten billion dollars annually; in Britain, the cost is estimated at £1,000 million. But what *is* pain?

Generally speaking, pain progresses from an awareness to a discomfort. It may then intensify until it dominates the senses, and finally explode into agony. For more than 2,000 years men have tried to define it, yet the mechanism by which it is produced is still not fully understood. Ever since he trod for the first time on a flint, fell out of a tree, or screamed as a carnivore's teeth ripped into his flesh, man has known pain. So has his mother in giving birth to him.

Pain divides itself broadly into two types: that which is caused from outside and that which starts within. But primitive man believed (and, indeed, natives in some parts of the world *still* believe) that *all* pain came from the outside. It could be caused, they believed, not only by thorns and arrows, clubs and fire, but by evil spirits (hence the dependence of primitive peoples on witch doctors). One view was that pain represented the spirit of another man, either dead or dying, seeking to enter a new body; or that it was the work of gods. In either case, the witch doctor was considered the only person able to give protection against pain. He could either supply potential victims with spells and charms – barriers through which it was said to be impossible for a restless spirit to penetrate – or he could placate the gods.

The early idea that pain was purely an outside force is sustained in the Bible. The prophet Job (Job 6:4) blames his pain on the 'arrows of the Almighty . . . within me'. David (Psalm 38) requests: 'O Lord, rebuke me not in thy wrath; neither chasten me in thy hot displeasure. For thine arrows stick fast in me and thy hand presseth me sore.'

The ancient Egyptians thought that pain entered through the left nostril or left ear. Any pain which did not have an immediate explanation (like a cut or a bruise, or the pricking of a splinter) was ascribed to a demon god (Seth and Sekhmet were the favourites). Spells were widely used, in addition to herbal remedies, and it was thought possible for a demon causing the pain to leave the body either in a sneeze, a good sweat, a load of vomit or dissolved in urine. The Assyrians also believed that pain was caused by intrusion from outside. Toothache, for example, was ascribed to worms getting into the teeth.

The Egyptians, Assyrians and Babylonians had no concept of the importance of the brain in recognizing pain. To them the organ which mattered was the heart. When a king was embalmed, his heart was carefully preserved but his brain was thrown away. It is to a Greek, a thousand years later, that the credit for first recognizing the brain as the centre of all sensation must go. His name was Alcmaeon, and he called the brain 'the sensorium'.

Alcmaeon was a pupil of Pythagoras. He noticed that if you banged an eye, you 'saw' flashes in the head. He attributed this to fire entering the eye and going to the brain. He attributed smell to solid particles entering the nose and travelling up ducts to the brain. Taste he described like this: 'It is with the tongue we discover tastes. For this being warm and soft dissolves the sapid particles by its heat, while by the porousness and delicacy of its structure it admits them into its substance and transmits them to the sensorium.' He did not actually link pain with the brain, but he did suggest that it was the seat of all sensation.

Plato, in similar vein, looked on the whole body as composed of atoms. Outside agents which produced pain, such as fire, were composed of sharper atoms. The sharper atoms cut into the softer body atoms and the information was communicated along blood-vessels to the soul. So a person felt 'pain when they (the atoms) suffer alteration, and pleasure when they are restored to their original state'.

In *Timaeus*, Plato wrote: 'All those parts which undergo violent alterations and are restored gradually and with difficulty to their original condition produce the greatest pains, as occurs with burnings and cuttings of the body.'

Plato was aware of the existence of the brain. He was aware of the spinal cord. But he was unaware of any central nervous system. It was not for another 600 years – not until a Greek called Galen started cutting open the bodies of animals – that the existence of a network of nerves leading to the brain was finally disclosed.

A WISE OLD GREEK

Galen was born in Pergamum, the capital of Asia Minor, in AD 130. He started studying medicine at the age of sixteen. Two years later he went to Smyrna to attend lectures given by a celebrated physician named Pelops. In search of more knowledge, he moved around other medical centres in Greece, Phoenicia, Palestine, Crete, Cyprus and Alexandria, before finally settling in Rome.

As a result of his observations, Galen relegated the heart to the status of a mere pump. The head he considered primarily to be a mount for the eyes. But the brain and the senses, in his view, were linked to different parts of the body by a network of nerves.

There were 'hard' nerves and 'soft' nerves, according to Galen. 'Hard' nerves were motor nerves; in other words, they controlled movement. 'Soft' nerves conveyed sensations. He believed that the two types of nerve actually served different parts of the brain, and he described how certain parts of the brain seemed softer than others.

Each organ in the body, according to Galen, had its own supply of nerve, artery and vein, in varying quantity. Not only could nerves feel or control; they could also learn by experience.

'Nature', he wrote in *De Usu Partium*, 'indeed has had a triple end in view in the distribution of nerves: she wished to give sensibility to organs of perfection, movement to organs of locomotion, and to all the others the faculty of recognizing the experience of injury. The third aim of Nature in the distribution of nerves is the perception of that which can cause harm.' In other words, pain.

If living things did not have this, he reasoned, they would soon die. He cited the example of pain in the intestines. Without it, he pointed out, we would be unaware that noxious substances were piling up inside us, trying to corrode, ulcerate or rot. Pain spurred us to get rid of these noxious substances before they could do damage.

Galen backed up his theories, wherever possible, by experimentation. He wrote a manual of dissection (*De Administrationibus Anatomicis Dissectorum*) describing many of his experiments on animals. In one section, he gives a graphic account of surgery on a new-born pig in which he describes how sensation could be affected by cutting through different parts of the spinal cord. Later, in *De Locis Affectis*, he reveals a more precise understanding of the origin of many nerves branching off from the spinal cord.

> Dissection has shown us that in the case of all parts of an animal below the neck that are moved voluntarily, the motor nerves originate in the so-called spinal marrow. You have also seen in dissections that the nerves which move the thorax originate in the spinal cord at the neck, and again it has been pointed out that transverse incisions which completely cut the cord destroy the sensation and mobility of all parts of the body situated below, since the spinal cord receives from the brain the faculties of sensation and voluntary movement. You have also seen in dissections that transverse incisions of the cord which stop at the centre do not paralyse all the lower parts but only those situated on the same side as the incision – i.e. those parts on the right, when it is the right portion of the cord which is cut, and those parts on the left when it is the left portion that is cut.
>
> Clearly then, when there is a condition at the origin of the cord which prevents the powers of the brain from reaching the cord, all the parts situated below, with the exception of the face, will be deprived of movement and sensation. . . . One who knows by dissection the origin of nerves that pass to each part will be better able to cure each part, deprived of sensation and movement.

Galen describes the case of a Syrian teacher of rhetoric who came to Rome to be treated for partial loss of sensation in his two little fingers. The man also had practically no sensation at all in half of the middle finger of his left hand. The Roman doctors had been unable to do anything for him, so he went to Galen. 'When I saw him,' Galen records,

> . . . I asked him about everything that had happened to him previously, and heard among other things that he had fallen from his carriage while travelling and had suffered a blow at the upper part of the back. This part had quickly become better but the loss of sensation in the fingers had gradually become worse. I ordered that the medicaments which his doctors had applied to his fingers be applied to the part where the blow had been received. In this way he was quickly cured.

He adds: 'The doctors do not even know that there are special nerve-roots which are distributed over the skin of the entire arm and to which the arm owes its sensation. . . .'

Galen was, perhaps, the first man to declare emphatically that the causes of pain may originate just as easily within as without. Among the internal causes of pain, he lists pulsation of the arteries and dyscrasia – an alteration in the balance of the 'humours' (the 'humours' were blood, phlegm, yellow bile and black bile, and a correct balance of these was thought necessary for good health). Dyscrasia he considered capable of triggering pain by means of pressure or tension.

Galen was centuries ahead of his time. His cardinal error – if it can be called an error – was in refusing to accept, as philosophers previously had asserted, that the soul was immortal. Indeed, he went so far as to suggest a close link between the so-called 'soul' and such banal conditions as intoxication by drink or drugs. As a result, his work was considered anti-Christian. It was therefore suppressed by those fathers of the Christian Church into whose hands, for the most part, the practice of medicine then passed.

ARISTOTLE PROVED WRONG

During the fourteen centuries following the fall of the Roman Empire, the failure of mankind to acquire a clearer understanding of the nature of pain was largely owing to the influence of Aristotle. The failure to develop effective ways of suppressing it can perhaps be attributed to the legend of Jesus Christ.

Throughout the Middle Ages, the great monasteries built all over Britain became the sole centres of medicine, from which herbal remedies, along with philosophy and reminders about morality, were obtainable. One of these reminders was that Christ had suffered on the cross. Was it not right, therefore, that all men should experience suffering to some degree?

Aristotle was a heart man – that is to say, he postulated that the heart and not the brain was the seat of all sensation and intellect. Because there was no shortage of Aristotelian disciples – and because his disciples tended to believe that *everything* the master said was right – the concept of the heart being the central repository for pain gained widespread acceptance, especially amongst religious men (who also shared Aristotle's view of the immortality of the soul).

Literature of the Middle Ages is sprinkled with references to the heart being the source of all sensory perception. St Jerome, one of the four great doctors of the Western Church and perhaps the most erudite of the Latin Fathers, wrote (around the turn of the fourth century): 'The Soul is not, as Plato said, in the brain but in the heart, according to Christ.' And woe betide those who thought otherwise. But the Arabs – outside the influence of Christianity – *did* think otherwise. A Persian physician glorying in the name of Abu-Ali

Al-Husain Ibn Abdullah Ibn Sina Avicenna, practising in the eleventh century, wrote a book called *The Canon of Medicine* in which he positioned the main receptor for pain in one of the cavities in the brain known as the anterior ventricle:

> Pain is one of the unnatural states to which the animal body, as a sensitive and living thing, is liable. Pain is sensation produced by something contrary to the course of Nature, and this sensation is set up by one of two circumstances: (a) a very sudden change of the temperature, or the bad effects of a contrary temperament; and (b) a solution of continuity.

What his 'solution of continuity' was need not concern us – it has no relevance to modern medicine – but the Persian *did* go on to describe fifteen different varieties of pain, including 'heavy pain' which, he said, was the kind of pain felt from 'an inflammatory process in an insensitive member such as the lung, kidney or spleen'.

'The weight of the inflammatory deposit', Abu-Ali Avicenna suggested,

> . . . drags on the tissues and surrounding sentient fascia and on its points of attachment. As the member is dragged on, the fascia and its point of attachment experience the sensation. The cause of the pain may be that a sentient member has had its sensation destroyed by disease, so that the weight is felt, but actual pain cannot be felt any longer.

The idea that the hub of all feeling lay in the anterior ventricle of the brain was subsequently accepted by three renowned surgeons of the Middle Ages – William of Saliceto, Guy de Chauliac and Henri de Mondeville Mondino. The latter's medical text book *Anathomia* certainly influenced the early thinking of Leonardo da Vinci, who was probably the next to take the search for an understanding of pain a step further.

Leonardo dissected many brains. He traced nerves leading from them and made wax casts of the cavities. He quickly discovered that the anterior ventricle – the front cavity favoured as the 'seat of sensation' by Avicenna – had no actual contact with the cranial nerves (the brain nerves involved in sight, smell, taste, breathing and much of the control of body muscles).

Leonardo therefore shifted the 'seat of sensation' from the anterior ventricle to a cavity further back, to the so-called middle or third ventricle, where most of the cranial nerves appeared to have their stalks. This he also pin-pointed as the 'seat of the soul'. All voluntary movement was controlled from there as well, 'at the place where all the senses come together, which is called the *senso commune*'. (Later he altered his opinion about the region of the brain involved in touch. That he allocated to the fourth ventricle, still further back.)

The nerves of touch, he considered, were the actual transmitters of pain, and he was well aware that part of the journey taken by a painful sensation led up the spinal cord. The fact that some regions of the body were more sensitive to pain than others intrigued him and in *Quaderni d'Anatomia* he wrote:

> In the movement of man, nature has placed all those parts in front which, on being struck, cause a man to feel pain: so it is felt in the shins of the legs, and in the forehead and nose. And this is ordained for man's preservation, for if such power of enduring suffering were not inherent in these parts, the numerous blows received on them would be the cause of their destruction.

THE SIXTEENTH AND SEVENTEENTH CENTURIES

Anatomy preoccupied many scientific minds in the sixteenth and seventeenth centuries as well as Leonardo's, and the period produced several refinements of the theory of sensation. Perhaps the most striking was the appreciation of the role of chemistry in bodily functions put forward by Paracelsus (1493–1541) and Van Helmont (1577–1649). The latter made a special study of the stomach and observed that the acidity of its contents could cause pain. He also noted that a painful injury to a limb could cause a person to be sick – owing to the pylorus (the circular muscle between the stomach and the duodenum) contracting – and so concluded that the pylorus rather than the brain was the centre of sensation in the body.

The French philosopher Descartes, on the other hand, believed that all consciousness stemmed from the 'pineal body', a small gland lying in the upper part of the mid-brain. 'Animal spirits' were also created there. Descartes (1596–1650) saw these as fine particles making up a kind of fluid which then flowed from the brain to all other parts of the body. He also believed that nerves were tubes containing a 'sort of marrow composed of a large number of exceedingly delicate threads starting from the proper substance of the brain'.

In 1644, Descartes published his famous work *L'Homme* in which – among many other things – he proposed a mechanism for pain based on the concept of nerve-threads leading to the brain. He published a sketch (*see figure*) showing what would happen if a person were to burn a foot. The caption read:

> If, for example, fire (A) comes near the foot (B), the minute particles of this fire (which as you know move with great velocity) have the power to set in motion the spot of the skin of the foot which they touch. By this means, pulling upon the delicate thread (CC) – which is attached to the spot of the skin – they open up, at the same instant, the pore (D, E) against which the delicate thread ends (just as by pulling at one end of a rope one makes to strike, at the same instant, a bell which hangs at the other end).

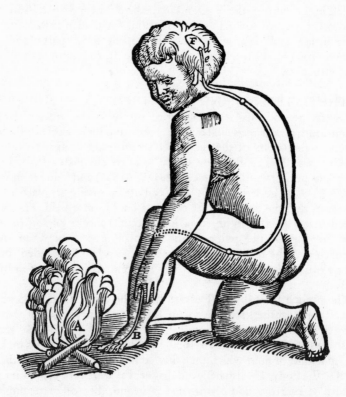

Involuntary movement: Descartes' idea of how impulses from the limbs reach the brain. Descartes believed all nerves to be hollow (ANN RONAN PICTURE LIBRARY).

A fine description of what we now call a 'nervous reflex'! Descartes also postulated that the degree of sensation felt by the person was in direct proportion to the tautness of his nerve-threads. In sleep, for example, the threads were totally relaxed, so the sleeper could feel nothing. Awake, the threads grew taut. Pleasure increased tension in them, and pain finally snapped them.

To support his theory that pain could only be appreciated in the pineal gland, he cited the case of a little French girl who had gangrene in her arm. Each time the arm was dressed, the doctor blindfolded the girl so that she could not see how bad it was. Eventually, a surgeon had to amputate it above the elbow. But she was not told what had happened. The dressings were put back to make it look as if the whole arm was still there, and the girl went on complaining 'for a long time' that she could still feel pain in her elbow, wrist and fingers. This was the first description of what is today termed 'phantom limb effect', and will be discussed more fully later.

THE EIGHTEENTH-CENTURY VIEW

The work of attempting to trace the paths of pain went on. At the start of the eighteenth century, a French anatomist named Vieussens tried frying brains in oil. He succeeded in showing up great fibre tracts leading to and from the brain but, like others of his time, he believed that sensations and limb movements were triggered and controlled by tiny particles of 'animal spirits' travelling up and down the nerves. Nerve 'juice' was put forward as another idea; the liquid was said to fill the nerves, which were still looked on as hollow tubes.

It was left to a Czech and a German to dispose finally of the myth that there was just one 'seat of sensation' – one *senso commune* – located solely in the brain, to which all individual nerves led. The Czech was called Georg Prochaska (1749–1820) and was profoundly impressed by what he saw when he executed a frog. The frog went on twitching and kicking even though its head and heart – and eventually its skin – were removed. Prochaska concluded that there was not one 'seat of sensation' but many, a veritable shower of reflex centres located all over the nervous system.

The German anatomist Soemmerring (1775–1830) performed dissections which led him to believe that nerves transmitted vibrations into the cerebro-spinal fluid – the liquid which does indeed fill cavaties in the brain and spinal cord – and that it was this fluid (of which an adult has about 130 cc) which was the 'seat of sensation'. But still no one had been able to unravel the mysteries of the spinal cord itself.

UNRAVELLING THE NERVES

The scene is Edinburgh, at the dawn of the nineteenth century. A young Scottish surgeon is operating on a puppy. The operation has no healing purpose and the surgeon finds it distasteful. Nevertheless, he perseveres, pausing from time to time, and walking over to a bench to make notes.

The puppy yelps, for anaesthetics are as yet unknown. As skilfully as possible, the surgeon cuts into its skull, exposing the brain and nerves leading away to the spinal cord. He touches some of them individually with his scalpel, observing how the puppy's limbs twitch – or fail to twitch – at each touch.

Eventually, when his dossier of notes is complete, he makes a sketch and puts the puppy out of its misery. Next day, he traces the sketch on to a plate and finally engraves it. Later he tells his brother: 'My new anatomy of the brain is a thing that occupies my head almost entirely.' The surgeon's name is Charles Bell.

Born in Edinburgh in 1774, Bell was the first man to explain that different nerves have different functions because they are linked to different parts of the brain. 'I consider the organs of the outward senses as forming a distinct class of nerves from the others,' he wrote in a letter to his brother George in 1809. 'I trace them to corresponding parts of the brain, totally different from the origin of the others.' He also observed three kinds of nerve: one carrying feeling, one controlling movement and a third carrying information to and from the vital organs, such as the heart, intestines or liver.

Bell made a vital observation about the spinal cord. In 1811, he wrote: 'The nerves of sense, the nerves of motion, and the vital nerves, are distinct throughout their whole course, though they seem sometimes united in one bundle.' In other words, all three different types of nerves were present in the spinal cord and connected to different areas of the brain. His experiments on living animals taught him that those which had their roots at the front of the spinal cord were definitely the ones involved in movement, but there is some argument over whether he similarly deduced that those with roots at the back were responsible for conveying feeling.

Bell caused pain to living animals, but he knew it was the only way to get a clearer understanding of the mechanism of pain in humans. In 1837 – six years after he was knighted and thirteen years after he became Senior Professor of Anatomy and Surgery at the College of Surgeons in London – he published a treatise called *The Hand*, in which he gave this view of pain:

Sensibility to pain varies with the function of the part. The skin is endowed with sensibility to every possible injurious impression which may be made upon it. But had this kind of degree of sensibility been made universal we should have been racked with pain in the common motions of the body; the mere weight of one part on another, or the motion of a joint, would have been attended with that degree of suffering which we experience in using or walking on an inflamed limb.

In what seems to be a side-swipe aimed at the Church, he adds: 'We perceive no instance of pain being bestowed as a source of suffering or punishment only.'

In another of his books, *System of Surgery*, he gives an interesting insight into pain-killing techniques used in operating theatres at that time:

The pain induced by operation may be lessened in different ways: by diminishing the sensibility of the system; and by compressing the nerves that supply the parts upon which the operation is to be performed. . . . As opiates are apt to induce sickness and vomiting, I seldom venture on giving them before an operation, unless the patient has previously been in the habit of using them. . . . It has long been known that the sensibility of any part may not only be lessened but even altogether suspended by compressing the nerves that supply it; and accordingly, in amputating limbs, patients frequently desire the tourniquet to be firmly screwed . . . finding that it tends to diminish the pain of operation.

He adds: 'The effect of this, however, is . . . inconsiderable.'

Sir Charles Bell's work was rivalled by that of a French contemporary, François Magendie. In fact, heated controversy broke out over which of the two first demonstrated the separate functions of the front (*anterior*) and back (*posterior*) nerves in the spinal column. The argument was eventually resolved by calling it thereafter 'the Bell-Magendie Law'.

The basis for our modern theory of sensation – and therefore for modern theories of pain – was further laid down by a German physiologist, Johannes Müller, who in 1842 propounded ten laws. These spelled out, amongst other things, the idea that the brain receives information about external objects only via the sensory nerves; that sensations can be triggered by internal causes as well as external; and that each organ of sense has its own nerves with 'its own peculiar quality, or energy'. Müller wrote:

Sensation is a property common to all the senses; but the kind of sensation is different in each: thus, we have the sensation of light, of sound, of taste, of smell and of feeling or touch. By feeling and touch we understand the peculiar kind of sensation of which the ordinary sensitive nerves generally – as the trigeminal, vagus, glosso-pharyngeal and spinal nerves – are susceptible. The sensations of itching, of pleasure and pain, of heat and cold, and those excited by the act of touch in its more limited sense, are varieties of this mode of sensation.

Müller's concept that each organ of sense – nose, eyes, ears, and so forth – was directly linked by nerves to an individual centre in the brain responsible for sensation, spurred him and his contemporaries to hunt for these centres. They started to look in the cortex – the outer layer of the brain – since it was the easiest to reach. Nerves leading from the eyes and the inner ears to the cortex were quickly identified, and it was assumed that the centres for sight and hearing lay, therefore, in that region of the brain. So convinced was one experimenter, Du Bois Reymond (1818–1896), that he suggested that if it were possible to connect the auditory nerve to the visual cortex, and vice versa, we should be able to see thunder and hear lightning. (Subsequent research has shown that the mechanism is not that simple and that the brain cortices are not wholly responsible for sensations of sight and sound.)

THE NINETEENTH-CENTURY VIEW

During the nineteenth century, techniques for investigating the human body improved dramatically. Microscopes became more powerful, and chemical procedures were devised for staining thin slices of tissue from different parts of the body so that they could be microscopically examined. The galvanometer was invented (1820) and this made it possible to standardize electrical shocks adminis-tered to the nerves of animals, so that reactions to pain could be more accurately measured. The full network of nerves in the body became more clearly defined, as did the mechanism of sensation.

A Frenchman called Charles Legallois made a significant contribu-tion towards understanding the nervous system by a series of operations on rabbits. Legallois was fascinated by the ability of decapitated creatures to go on living. He began removing sections of the brains and spinal cords of his rabbits to find out just how much of the nervous system was necessary for life.

In the course of these operations, he located the centre in the brain responsible for controlling breathing: it was a point at the very bottom, known as the *medulla oblongata*, where the brain joins the spinal cord. (There, too, lies the centre for controlling blood circulation.) He also found that breathing could be stopped by cutting nerves in two places in the spinal cord. From these observations, he deduced that various centres in the brain must act on other centres in the cord, which in turn controlled the muscles: in other words, that there was a hierarchy of sensation spread throughout the body and not simply confined to the head.

Legallois' work on removing parts of the brain and spinal cord provoked great public interest in France, where the Revolution had just extended the right of 'painless' execution by guillotine to the masses as well as the nobility. Could a chopped-off head *feel* anything? Parisians wondered. If Legallois' theories were correct, then it might be able to. And the idea gained some support when rumour swept Paris to the effect that the cheeks of a guillotined woman had blushed after decapitation when the executioner slapped them (the woman was Charlotte Corday, who had knifed Jean Paul Marat, the revolutionary leader, in his bath. The executioner is said to have picked up her severed head by the hair and publicly slapped both cheeks, producing a vivid reddening.)

In the latter half of the century, other research workers – notably a German called von Monakov – drew attention to the importance of the thalamus (a collection of nerve-cells in the forepart of the brain) as a kind of additional relay station for messages travelling between the sense-organs and their respective centres in the cortex. Von Monakov claimed that there were fifteen different zones in the thalamus linked to fifteen different regions of the cortex.

Next, another German – a physician named Max von Frey – did some remarkable work on the sensitivity of skin. In skin, he declared, there were four different types of sensing mechanism: one for touch, one for cold, one for warmth and one for pain. Each had its own 'receptors' located in different places in the skin. Previously, a number of other research workers had found a variety of specialized structures in skin to which they had given names like 'Ruffini end-organs', 'Krause end-bulbs' and 'Meissner corpuscles'. Von Frey knew also that there were two other very common types of structure, distributed liberally in the upper layers of skin – the so-called 'free nerve endings' and the fine fibres which entwine themselves around hair follicles.

Taking the five different types of structure as his starting point, he built some ingenious pieces of apparatus (two are still in use today). One is a pin on a spring, with which he was able to gauge the pressure needed to cause pain, and so map 'pain-spots'. The other is a piece of wood into which he fixed two-inch bristles of horsehair to map 'touch-spots'. He found literally thousands of pain-spots (there are in fact millions). Because they were so numerous he deduced that the 'free nerve endings' must be pain receptors. He deduced that 'Meissner corpuscles' must be touch receptors, since these were most frequently found at the tips of the fingers and in the palms of the hands. The fibres wrapped around hair follicles were touch receptors, too. 'Krause end-bulbs' he believed to be cold receptors, and 'Ruffini end-organs' receptors for warmth.

Von Frey was shrewd. Although recent research suggests that he was only partially right, his proposals became the basis for what is now called 'the specificity theory of pain': specific pain receptors transmit pain signals along specific pain fibres via a pain pathway to a pain centre in the brain. Some anatomists still accept this theory. But like so many instances in medical research when somebody comes up with a neat explanation or a pat answer, somebody else finds good reasons for disputing its veracity or even for rejecting it.

Opposition to the idea that there are paths of pain in the body came from an English neurologist called H. R. Marshall and a German physiologist, Ernst Heinrich Weber. Marshall claimed that pain was an emotion, not a sensation. He classed it along with pleasure. 'It appears to me', he wrote in the *Journal of Nervous and Mental Diseases* in 1894, 'that neurologists are wasting valuable labour in the search for "pain paths" in the spinal cord and the supposed nerve terminals, mediating some form of sensibility which under the conditions of examination are nearly always painful.' No pain centre had been located, he pointed out. Pain could be triggered by a whole host of things, whereas true sensations – smell, sight, hearing – had recognizable stimuli. Furthermore, pain could sometimes be imaginary. Ernst Weber claimed that pain was caused by a mixture of stimuli to the sensitive organs. *Any* sensory nerve could transmit it; it did not have to have a pathway of its own.

And so the argument went on and on. And to some extent it is still going on today.

THE 'GATE' THEORY

Up to the late 1960s, pain theorists drifted into one of two camps. One group held that pain had specific receptors and specific nervous pathways through the body – that the brain got the message 'pain' delivered on a plate. The other believed that *all* types of sensory receptor played a part in detecting pain – that they were *all* capable of producing coded patterns of signals for dispatch along nerves to

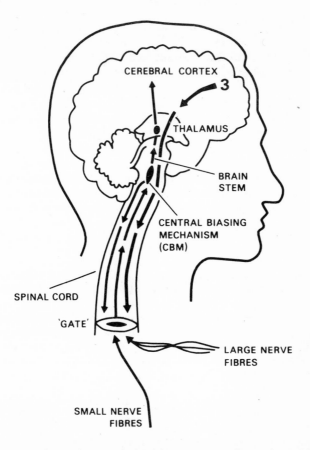

Pain experts have discovered that they can use electrical stimulation, acupuncture and hypnosis to relieve chronic pain. According to the gate control theory, these techniques produce relief by closing a hypothetical 'gate' in the spinal cord which blocks pain signals from reaching the brain.

1. Gentle electrical stimulation activates large nerve fibres that close the gate in the spinal cord, blocking pain signals to the brain.

2. Acupuncture stimulates small nerve fibres, sending impulses through the open gate that register in the brain as an acute pain of twirling needles. When the signals reach the central biasing mechanism in the brain stem, they trigger counter-impulses that travel down the spinal cord and close the gate against the chronic pain.

3. Hypnosis acts directly on the cerebral cortex, sending impulses down the cord and closing the gate.

the brain, and that the brain had to decide which patterns meant 'pain' and which did not.

Then, in 1965, Professor Patrick Wall (then at the Massachusetts Institute of Technology, now at London University) and Professor Ronald Melzack of McGill University, published a new theory of pain. They called it the 'gate' theory. They suggested that parts of the spinal cord acted as a gate to signals received from the skin, allowing only a selection to pass through to the brain.

In medical terms, they summed it up like this:

Stimulation of skin evokes nerve-impulses that are transmitted to three spinal cord systems: the cells of the *substantia gelatinosa* in the dorsal horn, the dorsal-column fibres that project towards the brain, and the first central transmission (T) cells in the dorsal horn. We propose that (1) the *substantia gelatinosa* functions as a gate control system that modulates the afferent patterns before they influence the T cells; (2) the afferent patterns in the dorsal-column system act, in part at least, as a central control trigger which activates selective brain processes that influence the modulating properties of the gate control system; and (3) the T cells activate neural mechanisms which comprise the action system responsible for response and perception. Our theory proposes that pain phenomena are determined by interactions among these three systems.

Figure A shows the factors involved in the transmission of impulses from peripheral nerve to T cells in the cord. If a single volley in large peripheral fibres arrives, there is a burst of rapid discharge in the cells followed by a turn-off. There is, at the same time, a negative dorsal-root potential produced by terminal depolarization and caused by *substantia gelatinosa* cell activity. If a small-fibre volley arrives, however, there is prolonged firing of the T cell which becomes more and more prolonged with each succeeding arriving volley, and there is a positive dorsal-root potential produced by hyperpolarization of the terminals, which we postulate is caused by inhibition of ongoing activity in *substantia gelatinosa* cells. Thus, volleys in large fibres are extremely effective initially but their later effect is reduced by the turning on of a negative feedback mechanism. In contrast, volleys in fine fibres activate a positive feedback mechanism which exaggerates the effect of arriving impulses. Figure A shows only presynaptic control, but presumably postsynaptic control mechanisms, not yet detected, also contribute to the observed input-output function. Furthermore, Taub and others have shown that descending impulses from the brain control the presynaptic mechanism, so that the ease with which impulses penetrate the cord-cells is determined both by the afferent activity and by central control processes originating in the brain.

Another aspect is that when pressure, temperature or chemical environments change, many fibres will start firing or will increase their activity. Even low-level stimuli will produce an increase in activity in fibres throughout the diameter spectrum. Since many of the larger fibres are inactive in the absence of change, a stimulus will produce a disproportionate relative increase of large over small fibre activity. The output of T cells, then, is determined by the number of active fibres and their rate of firing, by the balance of large and small fibre activity in the afferent barrage, and by the activity of central structures.

We propose that the signal which triggers the action system responsible for pain perception and response occurs when the output of T cells reaches or exceeds a critical level. There are two reasons for believing that pain results after prolonged monitoring of the afferent input by cells in the action system. First, threshold for shock in one arm is raised by a shock delivered as long as 100 milliseconds later to the other arm. Second, in pathological pain-states, delays of pain sensation as long as 35 seconds after stimulation cannot be attributed to slow conduction in afferent pathways. We suggest, rather, that there is a temporal summation or integration of the arriving barrage by central cells which finally results in pain perception and response when the integral exceeds a present level.

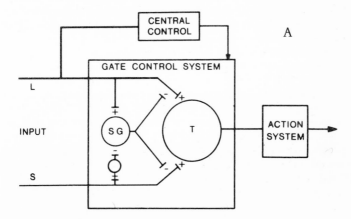

Schematic diagram of the gate control theory of pain mechanisms: L, the large-diameter fibres; S, the small-diameter fibres. The fibres project to the substantia gelatinosa (SG) and first central transmission (T) cells. The inhibitory effect exerted by SG on the afferent fibre terminals is increased by activity in L fibres and decreased by activity in S fibres. The central control trigger is represented by a line running from the large-fibre system to the central control mechanisms; these mechanisms, in turn, project back to the gate control system. The T cells project to the entry cells of the action system. +, excitation; − , inhibition

Wall and Melzack's 'gate' theory looked convincing. But soon research was suggesting that it was not the full story.

At the end of an International Symposium on Pain held at Rottach-Egern, Bavaria in 1969, Professor H. Hensel of the University of Marburg summed up the situation like this:

> In the further course of the discussion, the gate control theory (Melzack and Wall 1965) of pain was considered and criticism was expressed. Experimental findings were described (Eccles, Kostyuk and Schmidt 1962, Schmidt and Willis 1963, Eccles, Schmidt and Willis 1963, Franz and Iggo 1968, Jänig, Schmidt and Zimmermann 1968, Christensen and Perl 1970) which cannot be explained by the gate control theory, for example that isolated stimulation of C-afferents by current block as well as by cold block leads to depolarization and not to hyperpolarization of the primary afferent fibres, and likewise a painful thermal stimulation of a cat's paw leads to depolarization of the primary afferent fibres. Even if one found an experimental condition by which hyperpolarization of the primary afferent fibres occurred after stimulation from Delta-afferents or after stimulation from C-afferents, it is still probable that both of these fibre systems are not only responsible for pain conduction but also for other modalities. There is also no experimental support for the assumption that the cells of the *substantia gelatinosa Rolandi* are the cells of the reflex pathway of the presynaptic inhibition.
>
> The gate control theory is based on the particular hypothesis of continuous activity of those fibres which, coming from the skin, enter the posterior roots. This activity, discovered by Melzack and Wall in 1965, comprises the problem that the absence of any spontaneous activity is one of the particularly typical characteristics of the cutaneous afferent nerve-fibres. Furthermore, the original hypothesis is founded upon the assumption, for which there is so far almost no support, that the peripheral afferent C-fibres have a relatively uniform sensitivity to all types of stimuli.
>
> In addition, it has recently been proven that there are cells in the *substantia gelatinosa Rolandi* which apparently only have an input from high-threshold nociceptors; this also is against the gate hypothesis.
>
> Finally, the discussion dealt with the question whether pain or only indefinite false sensations develop by stimulation of the spinothalamic tract, whereas stimulation of the *funiculi posteriores* results in a precise projection of the periphery. It was also reported that in any case, no pain is produced by cutting through the spinothalamic tract and by electro-coagulation.

But Melzack and Wall were far from stumped. By 1973, they had revised their theory to take into account many of the objections. They revised it again in 1977 and Professor Wall pointed out (in *Brain*):

There were certain points in our original statement which seem to have been misunderstood and these need clarification. The diagram of mechanism we published had all the disadvantages of excessive clarity with its emphasis on the *substantia gelatinosa* and presynaptic mechanisms. The body of the paper mentioned other possible mechanisms. But it has seemed to some that the entire theory rested on the diagrammatic mechanism, which we shall see is not the case. Of course there have been many interesting discoveries since 1965 which need reviewing. Some of these new facts show that the data on which some of the theory was based was frankly misleading. Persistent inadequacy of technique still prevents an elucidation of mechanism.

He went on:

I would like to make a general restatement of the gate control theory in a form which I think is useful and defensible, and then to discuss the specifics in which we were clearly wrong in the light of subsequent work and the specifics which remain unknown.

1) Information about the presence of injury is transmitted to the central nervous system by peripheral nerves. Certain small diameter fibres (Ad and C) respond only to injury, while others with lower thresholds increase their discharge frequency if the stimulus reaches noxious levels.

2) The spinal cord or fifth nerve nucleus cells which are excited by these injury signals are also facilitated or inhibited by other peripheral nerve-fibres which carry information about innocuous events.

3) Descending control systems originating in the brain modulate the excitability of the cells which transmit information about injury.
    Therefore the brain receives messages about injury by way of a gate controlled system which is influenced by 1) injury signals 2) other types of afferent impulse and 3) descending control.

Peripheral nerves

In 1965, the literature on mammalian nociceptors was wrong and highly misleading because it appeared that adequate investigations of all types of peripheral nerve-fibres had been carried out. In the entire literature, only 20 myelinated fibres which could be called nociceptors had been described. The most complete study by Hunt and McIntyre [1960] found 7 nociceptors among 421 A fibres. This careful paper showed that their distribution of observed conduction velocities matched the observed distribution of fibre diameters, and therefore it seemed that they had adequately sampled the entire A population. Of the unmyelinated C fibres, Iggo had reported a few nociceptors

[1960]. However, it seemed possible that these might have been damaged by his dissection method because Douglas and Ritchie [1957] with their non-intrusive collision technique reported that all Ċ fibres responded to low-intensity stimuli. We reasonably concluded, 'These data suggest that a small number of specialized fibres may exist that respond only to intense stimulation [1965].' We knew, of course, from the extensive work from Adrian [1931] and Zotterman [1939] and Collins et al. [1960] that it had been repeatedly shown that stimulation of small diameter A and C fibres evoked pain, and we had to match this fact with the apparent rarity of pure nociceptors. The suggested solution was that an important part of the injury-signal was the high frequency and massed firing of those fibres, which had a wide dynamic range and responded to low-level stimuli and then increased their discharge-rate with more intense stimuli. These wide dynamic-range fibres also cluster in the smaller diameter range. Electrical stimuli which excited such fibres would then deliver a false injury-signal because of the combined spatial and temporal summation of the impulses on central cells.

The facts were wrong. The dissection and recording techniques had grossly biased the sampling in favour of larger fibres. We now know, thanks largely to the single fibre recordings in animals of Iggo and Perl and Burgess that substantial numbers of nociceptors exist [reviewed in Iggo, 1973]. The microelectrode technique of Vallbo and Hagbarth shows that these fibres also exist in man [Tjorebjork and Hallin, 1973, 1974; Van Hees and Gybels, 1972]. Some of these nociceptors become sensitized by prolonged or repeated noxious stimulation so that their threshold drops and they are excited by normally innocuous stimuli [Bessou and Perl, 1969], an observation which may be related to the primary hyperalgesia. The sensitization of nociceptors does not exclude them from being useful in signalling the presence of damage, since their receptors can be said to sense the continuing subliminal presence of injury which then reaches threshold when minor innocuous stimuli occur. Some terminals become less sensitive following injury, and these clearly do not signal the sequelae of injury or contribute to the pain suffered at some time after injury. The discovery of the class of nociceptive fibres is of obvious importance but as we stated [1965], 'This does not mean that they are "pain fibres" in that they must always produce pain and only pain when they are stimulated.' Nor does it mean that the high-frequency discharge of wide dynamic-range low-threshold fibres can now be neglected as playing no role in conveying to the CNS part of the message that injury exists.

Pathological peripheral fibres
The 1965 paper was written before the present explosion of information about the anatomical state of nerves in the peripheral neuropathies. We were highly influenced by the one detailed study available, on post-herpetic neuralgia [Noordenbos, 1959]. Weddell

had shown that intercostal nerve biopsy specimens provided by Noordenbos had a preferential loss of large myelinated fibres, and Noordenbos had generalized from this observation to propose that the pain was a consequence of a loss of inhibition normally provided by the large fibres. We now know that loss of large fibres is not necessarily followed by pain. In Friedreich's ataxia [Dyck, Lambert and Nichols, 1971] there is just such a preferential large-fibre deficit without pain. I thought it might still be possible to defend the generalization for adults, since Friedreich's ataxia begins at a very early age and it is possible that spinal cord compensations occur during the development of the unusual afferent pattern. However, this is no longer tenable since Thomas *et al.* 1971 showed that the polyneuropathy of renal failure in adults is not associated with complaints of pain although there is preferential destruction of large fibres. Any attempt to correlate the remaining fibre diameter spectrum with the symptomatology of neuropathies is no longer possible, as is apparent in recent reviews [Dyck, Thomas and Lambert, 1974; Thomas, 1975]. All combinations have been reported. For example, Fabry's disease is associated with a loss of small myelinated fibres and pain [Kocen and Thomas, 1970] but one hereditary sensory neuropathy [Schoene *et al.* 1970] is associated with a loss of myelinated fibres, preserved C fibres and analgesia. In an attempt to make sense of this chaos, Dyck, Lambert and O'Brien [1976] have introduced the dynamic factor of the presence of ongoing degeneration as well as the static existence of some particular fibre spectrum at the time of biopsy. Of their 72 patients with peripheral neuropathy, pain was present in 19 of 25 patients with acute fibre degeneration and only in 5 of 34 patients with other types of degeneration. Their conclusion is less impressive when one notices that 12 of the 19 patients with pain and acute degeneration had only 'a slight degree of pain, not a chief complaint, and analgesics were not used'. However, it does seem reasonable to conclude that fibre diameter alone is not enough or is completely irrelevant to explain the origin of pain in the neuropathies. How can this be? One possible answer is that the biopsy has not sampled the relevant region of nerve. In *tabes dorsalis*, the peripheral fibre spectrum is normal in spite of pain problems [Dyck *et al.* 1971], since the disorder is central to the dorsal root ganglion. In experimental neuromas of the rat sciatic nerve, the fibre spectrum of the parent sciatic nerve-fibre is almost normal, but only the small myelinated afferents and the unmyelinated afferents conduct impulses from the neuroma [Devor and Wall, 1976]. An anatomical study of the neuroma does not permit a statement of the diameter of the parent fibres which give rise to conducting fine sprouts that make up the neuroma. This leads to a further problem in interpreting a biopsy spectrum, since one cannot know that an observed fine fibre is not connected to a larger fibre, or what are the central connections of the observed fibre, or what are the properties of its peripheral receptor.

Obviously anatomy does not predict physiology. Intact fibres may be completely or partially blocked. Furthermore, as implied by Dyck *et al*. 1976, degenerating fibres may become spontaneously active or easily excited. Diamond [1959] showed that regenerating fibres become sensitive to acetyl choline. Wall and Gutnick [1974] showed that fibre sprouts within a neuroma are spontaneously active, pressure-sensitive, silenced by repetitive antidromic invasion and sensitive to noradrenaline. Evidently, degenerating, sprouting and regenerating fibres have unusual impulse generation and conduction properties. It might be thought that recording from single fibres in patients with neuropathies would resolve these issues but this is not entirely true because, like the biopsy, only one area is observed and the central destination of an observed impulse is not known. It is evident that we are unfortunately almost as free to speculate about the cause of pain in neuropathies now as we were in 1965, because the cause is unknown.

Cord cells responding to injury

Since only a partial survey of spinal cord cells had been carried out by 1965, we predicted the existence of injury-detecting cells and gave them the non-committal name of T cells. Now that many more cells have been recorded, one must first ask what are the criteria by which cells will be labelled as being concerned with pain mechanisms. Those committed to specificity theory consider only cells responding to injury and to no other stimuli. I take a more conservative approach and consider all cells responding monosynaptically to nociceptive afferents. Some would require that candidate cells must send axons into the contralateral ventral white matter. This is an unrealistic requirement, since peripherally-evoked pain recurs some weeks or months after anterolateral cordotomies [White and Sweet, 1969]. Some would even require that the cells must project to the thalamus, an even more unrealistic requirement in view of the abysmal failures of thalamotomies for the chronic relief of pain [White and Sweet, 1969]. It is not even necessary that the cells should project into long-running pathways, since it has been known since Schiff that bilateral and polysynaptic pathways can mediate pain [Basbaum, 1973]. It would be ideal if one could correlate the firing of cells with behaviour evoked by strong stimuli to determine the necessary if not sufficient conditions for the evocation of pain, but no such experiments are available. Similarly, no chemical or surgical blockade succeeds in permanent abolition of pain unless a complete disruption of projection pathways is achieved. Therefore these manoeuvres do not yet provide experimental evidence for selecting which cells or axons are crucial. A novel method introduced by Mayer, Price and Becker [1975], in which stimulus parameters needed to evoke pain and to stimulate particular types of cells are compared, offers a way of identifying cells involved in pain. What are the candidate cells?

1) Marginal cells, Lamina 1: Cells exist in this lamina which respond only to nociceptive afferents and to no others [Christensen and Perl, 1970]. Some of these project into contralateral ventral white matter, and some of these even as far as the thalamus [Dilly *et al*. 1968; Trevino *et al*. 1973; Kumazawa *et al*. 1975]. One must warn that such cells have been detected by these skilled and hard workers in very small numbers; an average of only two cells responding specifically to a nociceptive input have been recorded from each experimental animal. It would seem premature to adopt these cells as all that is necessary to explain pain mechanisms, as Kerr [1976] has done. They exist in a population of cells, most of which receive convergences from many types of peripheral afferent [Wall, 1968]. This fact warns one that one should be cautious in attributing one and only one function to a particular cell, since as we shall see, the degree of convergence is under control of other afferents and descending systems, and is also dependent on the activity of segmental interneurons. Furthermore, these cells do not match a number of simple expected correlations between their firing and pain behaviour. A powerful substance such as bradykinin does not excite them, and their discharge is not prolonged following injury [Christensen and Perl, 1970].

2) Lamina 5 cells: There are large numbers of cells in lamina 5 which respond to both myelinated and unmyelinated nociceptive afferents [Wall, 1967]. They respond to injury and to analgesic substances [Besson *et al*. 1972]. Their response to injury is decreased in the presence of narcotics and anaesthetics [reviewed by Mayer and Price, 1976]. Some have cutaneous receptive fields, while some receive high threshold afferents from muscle and others from viscera [Pomeranz *et al*. 1968]. In addition to their response to nociceptive afferents, most of these cells also respond to low-threshold afferents. Their receptive fields are therefore complex [Hillman and Wall, 1969]. The most dramatic of these convergences of high- and low-threshold afferents are on those cells which respond to high-threshold visceral afferents and also to low-threshold afferents from skin [Pomeranz *et al*. 1968]. The existence of these low-threshold excitatory convergences exclude these cells as candidates if complete specificity is required, but includes them if one wishes to explain such phenomena as hyperaesthesia, where light stimuli increase pain. Some of these cells project to opposite ventral white matter and some to thalamus [Trevino *et al*. 1973]. The papers of Mayer, Price and Beecher [1975] and Price and Mayer [1975] show that cells of this type are strong candidates for playing a role in pain evoked in man by stimulation of the ventro-lateral cord.

3) Other cells: A system of cells responding to intense peripheral stimulation and conducting slowly along the core of the spinal cord, medulla and mid-brain was described by Collins and Randt [1960]; no single-unit recordings have yet been made. It must be warned that recording methods still do not allow an exhaustive sampling of spinal cord cells. Therefore it may be that crucial populations of small cells remain undetected. One obvious group of small cells which have until very recently resisted recording are those in *substantia gelatinosa*. Heimer and Wall [1968] showed that final afferents terminate on these cells in cat and rat. Kumazawa and Perl [1977] have shown that cells in this region in monkey respond to nociceptive C afferents. Our own unpublished work on cat shows that there are several types of cells in *substantia gelatinosa*, many of which respond to low-threshold afferents. The anatomy of the region shows that cells only project over very short distances [Szentagothai, 1964]. Therefore they might only play a local segmental role in modulating the transmission of impulses from arriving afferents to cells which project over long distances [Wall, 1962]. However, it is also possible that they play a role in pain mechanisms as a system of multiple chains of short projection cells, as suggested by Noordenbos [1959]. A continuous column of spinal cord grey matter is not essential for the perception of pain, since cases of severe syringomyelia have been seen with complete obliteration of some segments of grey matter but preservation of white matter and of pain sensation. However, it is quite possible that short loops of axons extend from grey to white to grey matter, and thereby bypass the interrupted continuous column of grey matter in such cases.

Do peripheral afferents inhibit the cells excited by nociceptive afferents?
An essential feature of our hypothesis was that cells excited by injury afferents would be inhibited by low-threshold afferents. Subsequent discoveries have fully supported this aspect of the theory. Cervero et al. [1976] show that the discharge of the lamina 1 cells which are excited by noxious heating or by electrical stimulation of the A delta and C cutaneous afferents) are inhibited by electrical stimulation of the large (group 2) cutaneous myelinated afferents. An essential feature of the organization of lamina 5 cells is that they possess an inhibitory surround receptive field which is activated by low-threshold afferents [Hillman and Wall, 1969]. From the excitatory centre of the receptive field, low-threshold afferents evoke an excitation followed by a prolonged period of inhibition. Since the low-threshold large-diameter myelinated afferents send collaterals rostrally in the dorsal columns, it is not surprising that dorsal column stimulation also inhibits lamina 5 cells [Hillman and Wall, 1969]. Foreman et al. [1976] show that this inhibition is produced in the response of spinothalamic tract neurons in primates by stimulation of the dorsal columns. Electrical stimulation of bundles of axons is, of course, a crude, often misleading, manoeuvre, since it bypasses the specificity of input from different terminals, it fails to initiate the natural temporal pattern of impulses, and it smears the differing effects which depend on the spatial origin of the fibres. In spite of this

crudity, electrical stimulation of peripheral nerves or dorsal columns partially imitates the inhibition of lamina 5 cells which can be produced by discrete light-pressure stimuli in spatially specific parts of the cells' receptive fields. All of the candidate cells which respond to injury and which have been tested for their response to low-threshold afferents have been shown to be inhibited.

What is the mechanism of the afferent inhibition?

Melzack and I proposed as a secondary hypothesis that the gate control might be operated by a presynaptic mechanism, but we also stated that postsynaptic mechanisms could also operate. In the diagram we made the error, for the sake of simplicity, of showing only a presynaptic mechanism, and a number of critics including Nathan have missed what was written in the text and have assumed that we proposed only a presynaptic mechanism, and furthermore that the whole theory rested on this mechanism. The theory in fact rests on the presence of inhibitions and facilitations, and these are undoubted. The question of whether these are pre- or postsynaptic is secondary but, of course, of considerable interest. Hongo *et al.* [1968] showed that there were undoubted signs of postsynaptic inhibition, and this work remains the only definite identified location of an inhibition. This does not exclude the possibility that presynaptic inhibition might not also operate. It is certain that there are depolarizations of the terminals of the afferent fibres. These generate the dorsal-root potentials and the lowering of threshold of the afferent fibre's terminals. The mechanism by which this afferent depolarization occurs remains in doubt. The depolarization is very loosely coupled with an inhibition of transmission from afferents to interneurons. We had suggested that these presynaptic changes were associated with a block of transmission from the entering fibres into the terminal arborization [Howland *et al.* 1955], and Eccles [1964] had proposed that a depolarization of terminals would result in a decrease of transmitter release. Both of these suggestions are based on circumstantial evidence and still lack proof in the mammal. Neither of these proposals excluded that there was not a concomitant and perhaps predominant postsynaptic change which explained the observed inhibition. I wish to emphasize that an undoubted presynaptic depolarization occurs; its origin is unknown; it roughly coincides with an inhibition; however, for the only candidate cells which have been examined, there are also postsynaptic changes. Therefore, it is still a matter of speculation to propose the origin of the observed inhibition. Unlike some invertebrate synapses, the mammalian dorsal horn still contains synaptic interconnections too small and too intricately interwoven to allow definite causal mechanisms to be demonstrated which explain observed input-output functions.

It was proposed that the cells of *substantia gelatinosa* played a role in the modulation of transmission. Their anatomical location with short running axons interposed in the junction region of afferents and dendrites made them suitable for this role. Further details of this anatomy [Kerr, 1975] emphasize this possibility but do not help in the pre- or postsynaptic controversy. A positive physiological reason for their inclusion was the observation that the Lissauer tract, which interconnects the cells of *substantia gelatinosa*, was capable of spreading the primary afferent terminal depolarization from one segment to another [Wall, 1962]. Since that time Denny-Brown *et al.* [1973] have given more substantial reasons for involving the Lissauer tract and therefore the *substantia gelatinosa* in the regulation of the effectiveness of afferent impulses. They showed that the dermatome subserved by an isolated dorsal root, as tested by behavioural reaction to cutaneous stimulation, was greatly expanded if the Lissauer tract, entering the innervated segment, was sectioned. Exciting and important as this observation is, it must be pointed out that it cannot tell how the *substantia gelatinosa* cells are involved in the pathway from the dorsal root to the observed motor responses. It is clear that techniques will have to be developed to modify independently the action of *substantia gelatinosa* cells and to record from them before proceeding to test how they are involved in the excitability of reflex areas or sensory transmission. All of the work since 1965 shows that cord cells responding to injury are subject to inhibitions of peripheral origin, but the mechanism remains obscure.

Facilitations

There has been remarkably little progress on the subject of facilitation as distinct from excitation. The reason is a technical one. The cells under discussion are excited by small diameter afferents which conduct slowly, and the action potentials in the fibres are difficult to record. In certain favourable situations, cells may respond only to a particular group of small afferents, as in the case of lamina 5 cells responding to the splanchnic nerve [Pomeranz *et al.*, 1968] or the lamina 1 cells [Christensen and Perl, 1970]. This allows a satisfactory timing of the first discharge of the cell and a proof that it is responding, probably monosynaptically, to the leading edge of the arriving slow volley. However, many of these cells then respond repetitively and it is not easy to prove if these subsequent responses of the cell are due to excitation by trailing slowly-conducted impulses in the afferent volley, or are produced by some reverberation within the cell, or by the action of some nearby cells. We proposed in 1965 that a source of long-lasting facilitation was a hyperpolarization of the terminals of afferent fibres produced by the arrival of volley in small diameter afferents. There was, for a time, a controversy as to whether this primary afferent hyperpolarization existed at all, but it now seems generally agreed that hyperpolarizations exist but are not necessarily associated with the arrival of afferent volleys in small nociceptive afferents [reviewed, Wall, 1973]. In earlier work [Wall, 1959], I gave reasons to suggest that the prolonged repetitive firing of dorsal horn interneurons was neither a property of the afferent volley nor of the responding transmitting cells, and therefore must be attributed to some other mechanism. For the reasons stated, this problem has not been a major target of investigation although it will be important in understanding pain mechanisms, particularly in those situations of hypaesthesia where slowly repeated stimuli result in a slow wind-up of sensation reminiscent of the wind-up of cell response [Mendell, 1966]. These gradually escalating pains are evoked by such slowly repeated stimuli that each stimulus must leave behind it a period of facilitation which exaggerates the effect of the subsequent stimulus [Noordenbos, 1959] and cannot be examined by a dispersion of the arrival-time of the afferent volley.

Are the injury detecting cord cells subject to descending control?

An essential feature of the gate-control hypothesis was that the cord cells which received nociceptive afferents would be under descending control, and this has proved to be the case in all cells so far examined. In the decerebrate animal, a powerful tonically-active inhibitory system within the pons and medulla projects into the dorsal horn. This system inhibits the effects of cutaneous and visceral afferents on dorsal horn neurons. This was first noticed by Sherrington and Sowton [1915] in comparing reflex activity in spinal and decerebrate animals. Wall [1967] showed that it was possible to follow the activity of single cells before, during and after the cold block of a segment of spinal cord which blocked the descending inhibition in cerebrate animals. Cervero *et al.* [1976] located 46 cells in the marginal layer, lamina 1, 35 of which responded only to nociceptive afferents and 11 responded to sensitive mechanoreceptors as well as to nociceptors. When the spinal cord was cold blocked, both types of cell became more excitable. The lamina 5 cells have been studied in more detail, Wall [1967], Hillman and Wall [1969]. In the decerebrate state, their receptive fields are smaller, the ongoing activity is less, the inhibitory areas are more effective and the response to injury is smaller than in the spinal state. Small lesions and microelectrode stimulation show that this inhibitory pathway descends in the dorsolateral white matter. Other descending systems such as the pyramidal tract [Fetz] and vestibulospinal system [Erulkar *et al.* 1966] also control dorsal horn interneurons. One of these systems descends indirectly from the mid-brain periaqueductal grey, PAG. Stimulation of this area produces a profound analgesia in animals and man [Reynolds, 1969; Mayer and Liebeskind, 1975; Adams, 1976]. The same stimulation inhibits the response of lamina 5 cells to noxious stimuli [Oliveras *et al.* 1974]. The behavioural analgesia must be produced by a descending inhibitory system, since unilateral section of the dorsolateral white matter in rat thoracic cord abolishes the analgesia in the ipsilateral hind leg while leaving the other three limbs analgesic [Basbaum *et al.* 1976, 1977].

The descending pathway seems to relay in the cells of the nucleus *raphe magnus* [Fields *et al.* 1977; Basbaum *et al.* 1977] and to be dependent on monoaminergic transmitters [Engberg *et al.* 1968; Akil and Liebeskind, 1975].

The effect of the success of transcutaneous nerve stimulation on the gate control theory

The most obvious prediction of the gate control theory was that stimulation of large-diameter peripheral nerve-fibres should raise the threshold for detecting injury in the region served by the stimulated nerve. Sweet and I [1967] immediately proceeded to test this with considerable trepidation, since we did not know if the predicted threshold rise would be significant or, worse, if the excitatory effects in man would overwhelm the inhibitory ones. We were well aware of the fact that electrical stimulation of peripheral nerve produces an abnormal concatenation of spatial and temporal convergences of peripheral afferents on to central cells. However, we hoped that the artificial barrage produced by low-level peripheral nerve stimulation would have an overall inhibitory effect on human cord cells, as it does in the cat. The predicted rise of threshold was shown to occur in normal subjects [Higgins, Tursky and Schwartz, 1971; Satran and Goldstein, 1973; Campbell and Taub, 1973]. In certain patients with chronic intractable pain, the effect of transcutaneous electrical stimulation is sufficiently powerful for therapeutic use. In a series of 336 cases with peripheral disease reported by Long and Hagfors [1975], 129 gained full pain relief from counterstimulation, while of 60 cases with central disorders only 2 responded. In a survey of over 3,000 patients at various centres, 25–30 per cent of patients previously incapacitated completely by chronic pain were more or less completely relieved of pain [Long and Hagfors, 1975]. 11 of 30 chronic severe cases of post-herpetic neuralgia responded satisfactorily over long periods of time to transcutaneous stimulation [Nathan and Wall, 1974].

The theory proposed that stimulation of large-diameter afferents would, on average, raise the threshold of central cells by increasing inhibition. In spite of the apparent support given to this proposal by the clinical results, I was from the beginning cautious about this conclusion for two reasons. One was the observation that certain types of pathological pain would completely disappear while leaving the area normally sensitive to pin-prick and pinch [Lindblom and Meyerson, 1975]. This suggested that there was something special about these pains, the control which did not necessarily interact with 'normal' pain. The second reason was that some patients experience relief for hours after minutes of stimulation, while the inhibitions which we observed in animals only outlasted the stimulus for seconds.

Campbell and Taub [1973] proposed that the electrical stimulation was so intense that the peripheral nerves themselves were blocked. Using pulse-widths ten times those normally used and voltages five times higher, they presented possible evidence that peripheral nerves are blocked. Ignelzi and Niquist [1976] also show peripheral nerve-block in animals, but they appear to have applied the full current across sural nerve which is normally distributed across an entire leg. It has been known since the first man recovered from a bolt of lightning that intense electrical stimulation will block nerve, but can this be the explanation for the clinical results? The answer is No because if it were so the treated area should be anaesthetic, which it is not, and dorsal column stimulation should never work, although it does. Furthermore, in order to block a nerve with the intense currents used by Campbell and Taub, it is necessary to stimulate both large and small fibres before they block, and even when part of the nerve is blocked the stimulation continues on the edge of the block. If only peripheral block were to occur, the subject would be in intense pain during the onset of the block and while it was maintained. Since he is not, one must propose that some central inhibitory mechanism has been set off by the initial low-stimulus intensities used, and that this inhibition is sufficient to allow the subject to tolerate the subsequent barrage generated by the higher currents.

Worried by the discrepancy between the clinical results and our predictions in which the clinical relief over-fulfilled the prediction, Gutnick and I [1974 a & b] turned to examine the physiology of abnormal peripheral nerve. In rats, the sciatic nerve was cut and the end was placed in a tube so that the neuroma developed within the tube. Impulses were recorded in single dorsal-root fibres, the ends of which lay within the neuroma. The intact parent fibres which sprout to form the neuroma are almost entirely small-diameter fibres [Devor and Wall, 1976]. Many of these fibre terminals give rise to ongoing activity. We placed stimulating electrodes on the proximal intact nerve and, in imitation of therapeutic counterstimulation, a 100 Hz 0.1 m/sec square wave stimulation was applied. To our surprise, the antidromic invasion of the sensory terminals in the neuroma by the high-frequency train of impulses was followed by long periods of silence of the previous ongoing activity, and by long periods of insensitivity to electrical or mechanical stimuli. After a few seconds of tetanus, these neuroma terminals took minutes or hours to recover their previous sensitivity. If normal intact terminals are invaded by such a volley, they recover their excitability within seconds. It is evident that either the nerve-impulse generator mechanism or the transmission properties of axons in a neuroma have abnormal properties which fail to recover after high-frequency driving. If these abnormal properties exist in the membrane of human pathological peripheral axons, it may then be that part of the explanation for the effectiveness of electrical stimulation lies in the periphery rather than in the cord. However, one must stress that it is still necessary to postulate central inhibition as well as a possible peripheral mechanism, since otherwise it would be impossible to reach the required voltages of stimulation without inflicting intolerable pain. If the stimulating current is gradually raised during the application of surface stimulation with 100 Hz 0.1 m/sec square waves, a voltage is reached at which the subject feels a strong, buzzing, tingling sensation. If a short burst of stimuli at this voltage is applied without preconditioning, the result is intense pain. The reason for this difference is that the preceding low-level stimuli have produced central inhibition. The striking and long-lasting abolition of pain from damaged nerve by counterstimulation may therefore be due to a combination of central inhibition and peripheral inactivation. However it remains possible that such nerves generate unusual central patterns of response which are particularly easily inhibited by afferents.

Professor Wall summed up the revised 'gate' theory like this:

> In 1965, we proposed that the transmission of information about injury from the periphery to the first central cells was under control. The setting of this control or 'gate' was influenced by peripheral afferents, other than those which signalled injury. The 'gate' was also influenced by impulses descending from the brain. Subsequent work has fully supported and enlarged this view . . . . The mechanism by which impulses descending from the brain achieve control remains completely unknown, as is the role of the *substantia gelatinosa*.
>
> That a 'gate' control exists is no longer open to doubt. But its functional role and its detailed mechanism remain open for speculation and for experiment.

PAIN – AN EXPLANATION

While the scientific argument continues – and until somebody comes up with a better explanation – perhaps I may be forgiven for liking our present concept of the mechanism of pain to the structure of Britain's defences in the 1939–45 war.

A large number of outposts – mostly located around the perimeter, but some inland – is constantly on the alert for signs of trouble; each outpost is connected by telephone line to a headquarters; the regional headquarters is connected by a main trunk line to the seat of government in the capital, where all the major decisions are taken. At the first sign of invasion, a message is flashed along the line in code. The regional headquarters decides whether to pass it to higher authority. The government up top then decides – in the light of all the information available and all its experience of the past – whether to react to it or ignore it. Orders are sent out accordingly.

The ever-watchful outposts, in the case of the human body, are the so-called receptors. There are literally millions of them. They feel heat, cold and touch but not specifically – according to this latest theory – pain, although they do detect injury. The majority are located in the skin, although internal organs have them too. One count has put the total of heat receptors in the skin at 30,000, the cold receptors at 250,000 and the touch receptors at well over 3,000,000. Strangely enough, the surface of the brain – the roof over the seat of government, if you like – has none (at least, none has so far been discovered). In that sense, the analogy with wartime defences is inaccurate, for at least there were fire-watchers and Observer Corps posts on the roofs of government buildings during the Blitz!

The heart has comparatively few receptors. William Harvey, discoverer of the circulation of the blood, observed this in the seventeenth century. He relates in *De Generatione Animalium* how the then Viscount Montgomery's heir, Hugh, suffered a massive injury to his chest and arrived in London with a gaping hole 'open in his Breast, so that you might see and touch his lungs (as it was believed)'. Closer inspection revealed that it was not the young man's lungs which were visible but his heart.

> Therefore, [Harvey continues] instead of an Account of the Business, I brought the Young Gentleman himself to our late King, that he might see, and handle this strange and singular Accident with his own Senses; namely, the Heart and its Ventricles in their pulsation, in a young and sprightly Gentleman, without offense to him: Whereupon the King himself consented with me That the Heart is deprived of Sense of Feeling. For the Party perceived not that we touched him at all, but merely by seeing us, or by the sensation of the outward skin.

Harvey adds that the young Montgomery 'was not seriously inconvenienced by having this permanent opening in his thorax, and lived a very active life, fighting first for the King's authority in Ireland and afterwards against Cromwell'.

Receptors are minute detectors. Each has a slender filament of nerve leading away from it, like the telephone line in our wartime defence system. As soon as a receptor is stimulated, it sends off a message – a series of tiny pulses of electrical energy – down the nerve. The strength of these signals, it is believed, is in direct proportion to the stimulus detected.

The message (and other messages from nearby receptors) travels along the 'telephone line' at fantastic speed – sometimes nearly 400 feet per second.

The nerves converge first into bundles. The bundles converge into trunks. The trunks converge into the spinal column (the regional headquarters) and finally go to the brain. On the way, the messages are sampled. This is done in a region of closely-packed nerve fibres which runs the full length of the spinal column, on both sides. It is known as the *substantia gelatinosa*. It is what Wall and Melzack call their 'gate'.

The *substantia gelatinosa* seems to act rather like an intelligence officer at regional headquarters, sifting the coded signals and deciding which are important enough to pass on. It is thought to have the power to block off some of the information – to handle it itself without reference to higher authority. Thus if somebody tickles your foot, the *substantia gelatinosa* takes care of your reaction, sending out orders to muscles to jerk the foot away, without bothering the brain with the problem. On the other hand, if you step on a thorn, it will pass the information through to its superior.

'Cleared' information about heat and cold and touch is transmitted up the spinal cord, from the region known as the dorsal horn, along more nerve fibres to the head. Some of these nerve fibres lead directly to the thalamus (one of the cabinet offices in the seat of government) located in the fore-brain. These fibres are equivalent to the 'hot lines' or 'red telephones' in a modern defence headquarters. The majority of messages, however, are sorted in the *reticular formation*, a tangled skein of inter-connecting fibres located in the centre of the brain, near its base. This mess of nerves (equivalent to a whole department of Civil Servants or colonels) sorts out the information more thoroughly and then dispatches it, via any number of possible routes, to its final destination, the highest regions of the brain (seat of government) or cortices.

It is over the precise routes taken by patterns of information to the higher regions of the brain that most of the argument over the mechanism of sensation and pain still persists. Not all scientists yet accept that there is a 'gate' in the spinal cord. Some still insist on separate pathways for pain leading to the brain, and on specific 'pain receptors'.

Professor Melzack, however, insists:

> We now believe that receptor mechanisms are more compli-
> cated. There is general agreement that the receptors which
> respond to noxious stimulation are widely branching, bushy

networks of fibres that penetrate the layers of skin in such a way that their receptive fields overlap extensively with one another. Thus, damage at any point on the skin will activate at least two or more of these networks [*The Puzzle of Pain*, Penguin Educational, 1973].

Certainly, the way receptors handle different 'noxious' stimuli varies from place to place in the body. Jab a pin into your finger and you feel an immediate prick of pain: jab it into an intestine and you feel no pain; nor will you even if you slash the intestine with a knife. But an intestine *will* register pain if it is stretched or jerked.

Dr James Hardy, of the University of Pennsylvania Medical School, likens pain to a speedometer which 'measures the speed at which tissue damage is occurring: it tells you little about the seriousness of your injuries, but warns you how rapidly injury will proceed if you don't take action'.

Indeed, you could sit in a bath for six or seven hours with the water temperature around 112°F. – hot enough to cook your skin nicely – without feeling much pain: yet if you were to touch the back of your hand accidentally with a red-hot poker for even a fraction of a second you would feel intense pain. Undoubtedly, the rate of activity of receptors – and the numbers involved in an injury – are important factors in the body's assessment of pain. But they are not the whole story. . . .

THE MIND INTERVENES

The sea was flecking up into little 'white horses' as assault landing craft PA 34–18 moved in towards the beachhead at Anzio. Behind the silhouette of the sand-dunes, buildings in the town could be seen burning vigorously. A pall of smoke hung over the area. The twelve-inch German guns and rocket launchers had been silenced but there was still some sporadic machine-gun and rifle fire.

Medical orderlies were collecting up the bodies of the dead and wounded 'White Devils' – men of the 1st and 3rd Battalions, US Rangers who had spearheaded the assault on Anzio – from the more remote niches in the sand-dunes, where they had fallen to German bullets a short while previously.

PA 34–18 crunched into the shingle, its ramp went down and an officer ran forward. He headed up the beach towards a group of especially large sand-dunes, where a gang of soldiers was erecting a green marquee. Lt.-Col. Henry Beecher, US Army Medical Corps, quickly went across to a line of stretchers on which wounded soldiers were lying. What he saw then – and subsequently as he moved around the beaches – made him realize just how much pain is affected by one's attitude of mind.

Wounded GIs – some of them with hideous gaping wounds, others with whole limbs shot away – were lying almost contentedly in the sand. There was barely a moan from any of them – until, that is, a medical corpsman approached with a syringe. Then, in Dr Beecher's own words, 'most of them yelled like hell'.

Why? Why did the men accept the massive pain from their wounds but apparently fear the slight pain of the needle?

There was opportunity that night, after the forward hospital had been erected, to explore this further. Dr Beecher devised a questionnaire. 'As you lie there,' he asked each wounded man, 'are you having any pain?' If the answer was 'yes', the man was then asked: 'Is it slight pain, or moderate pain, or bad pain?' Finally he was offered something to relieve it 'if the pain is bad enough'.

10 out of the 225 patients had bullet or shrapnel wounds in the head, or were unconscious, and so they were excluded. But of the remaining 215, 69 (32.1%) claimed they felt no pain at all, 55 (25.6%) said they felt only slight pain, 40 (18.6%) admitted moderate pain and the remaining 51 (23.7%) were in great pain. Of those in pain, 157 (73%) did not wish to be given a pain-reliever. Why?

Dr Beecher comments: 'A badly injured patient who says he is having no wound-pain will still protest as vigorously as a normal individual at an inept venipuncture (injection). It seems unlikely, therefore, that the freedom from pain of these men is to be explained in the basis of any general decrease of pain sensibility.' Nor were the wounds of such a trivial nature as to be unlikely to cause pain: nearly half had abdominal wounds, nearly a quarter compound fractures and the rest either penetrating wounds or extensive injury to the flesh.

In his report in the *Annals of Surgery* (1946, no. 123, p. 76) Dr Beecher calls the whole affair 'puzzling', adding: 'A comparison with the results of civilian accidents would be of interest. While the family automobile in a crash can cause wounds that mimic many of the lesions of warfare, it is not at all certain that the incidence of pain would be the same in the two groups.' He adds:

Pain is an experience subject to modification by many factors: wounds received during strenuous physical exercise, during the excitement of games, often go unnoticed. The same is true of wounds received during fighting, during anger. Strong emotion can block pain. That is common experience. In this connection it is important to consider the position of the soldier: his wound suddenly releases him from an exceedingly dangerous environment, one filled with fatigue, discomfort, anxiety, fear and real danger of death, and gives him a ticket to the safety of the hospital. His troubles are about over, or he thinks they are. He overcompensates and becomes euphoric.

Dr Beecher goes on: 'Whether this actually reduces the pain remains unproved. On the other hand, the civilian's accident marks the beginning of disaster for him. It is impossible to say whether this produces an increased awareness of his pain, increased suffering; possibly it does.'

Dr Beecher also points out that many other factors than the sheer relief of qualifying for a Purple Heart and being removed from the battle may influence a wounded man's attitude to pain. He says:

The circumstances that have led to the wound may have been associated with anxiety; with emotional stress; with grief from the loss of friends; with fear; and these have often been exaggerated by the sights and sounds of prolonged combat, coupled with the physical discomforts of exposure to the weather, inadequate food and fluid intake, loss of sleep, exhaustion, as well as by pain. On top of all this, the newly wounded man suddenly has to face the consequences of his wound: his arm is injured – will he lose it? There is blood around his genitals – will he be impotent? That wound in his chest – is he going to die? Given half a chance, indications of great mental agitation come out in a rush, from men who have been lying quietly, often seemingly asleep.

Dr Beecher also suggests that the drug which was most widely used for relieving pain in battle in those days – morphine – may be entirely unsuitable for the treatment of certain types of wounded. Barbiturates may be better. He cites this example:

A husky 19-year-old soldier was wounded at the Anzio beachhead by a mortar shell. Five hours later he was brought into the nearest hospital with a meat cleaver-like wound cutting through the fifth to twelfth ribs near the vertebral column. He had bled a great deal (haemoglobin 9.5g; not yet completely diluted) and was cyanotic. Obsessed with the idea that he was lying on his rifle, he constantly struggled to get off the litter and complained bitterly of the 'pain'. Three attendants were necessary to keep him on the litter. Examination of the patient in any adequate sense was impossible. He appeared to be wild from pain. His wound supported such a belief. (Not only were eight ribs cut in two, and an open pneumothorax present, but later it was found that the lower lobe of his lung, the diaphragm, and one kidney had been lacerated by a broken rib-end.) He had had no morphine for at least four hours, and it was planned to give him more; but since the situation was confused, it was decided to give him 150 mg(2.5 gr.) sodium amytal by vein. This was done, and he at once quieted down and went to sleep. Obviously no morphine was needed.

The patient was rousable but remained quiet for the next hour, until he went to the operating room. During the quiet period he was examined, and catheterized, previously impossible, and found to have grossly bloody urine. Immediately after receiving the barbiturate, his colour improved strikingly, doubtless in part due to the cessation of great physical exertion and to the fact that instead of constantly yanking out his nasal oxygen tube it stayed in place, and his blood-pressure rose at once from 60 up to 80 mm. Hg systolic. Before the barbiturate was given, all agreed that the patient's condition was rapidly deteriorating; he turned for the better immediately after the amytal was given. The dose given would not have controlled pain. It is reasonable to conclude that his manic state was not due to pain.

Dr Beecher's observations stimulated interest afresh in the subject of pain 'threshold': in other words, the level at which an individual (a) feels pain and (b) wishes to do something about it. This may depend on many things. . . .

2

Mind over Matter

It is quite possible that a human may be able to feel pain from the seventh week after conception, as an embryo less than half an inch long. At that stage, the embryo has a beating heart, buds for limbs, a brain and spinal cord, but no experience of what is painful and what is not.

By the ninth week it has eyes and an inner ear, and the spine is beginning to move. Two weeks later, most of the organs needed for life have started to function. By the twelfth week it is fully formed; thereafter it merely grows and matures. By the end of the twenty-eighth week it is reckoned to be capable of leading a separate existence and can certainly respond to stimuli, even if unable to recognize them as painful.

It is hard to define the exact point at which an infant first reacts to pain. The business of being squeezed out through the mother's uterus results in a cry – the first of many in the early days of life – but that seems merely to be Nature's way of getting air into the lungs. It is known that acute hunger results in pain, and crying before feeding time – as early as the first week of life – may be an expression of that pain. Crying is part of a baby's natural daily existence – it is good exercise and does no harm. But the cries themselves vary. Some relate to thirst, others to temper; some are definite responses to 'noxious stimuli' like cold or heat or a skin rash, and it is these latter types which a mother learns quickly to recognize as the sound of her baby 'in pain'.

Some people are born insensitive to pain. They usually suffer frequent bruising, deep burns and numerous cuts and grazes as children, before they learn to be especially wary of injurious agents. They can even bite the tip off the tongue while chewing food, without realizing what they have done, and sometimes the smell of scorching flesh is their first warning of a severe burn.

The body normally responds to alarm signals which indicate pain in a number of ways. Blood which ordinarily circulates through the skin and abdominal organs is quickly re-routed to the brain, lungs and muscles. The heart beats faster and blood-pressure rises – both, apparently, in readiness to deal with the source of the pain. The liver secretes a reserve of sugar into the bloodstream – instant food for the muscles so that they can react – while chemical changes occur in the blood itself, giving it the power to clot more quickly so that a minimum is lost.

If the source of the pain is internal rather than external, a different set of protective responses is triggered. Blood-pressure may drop; nausea may begin, making the person in pain want to curl up – an excellent posture for recovery. But in a 'pain blind' person, the protective mechanism fails to jerk into action and the result may be – as with, say, appendicitis – that death can draw close before the gravity of the situation is realized.

Professor Melzack, in *The Puzzle of Pain*, cites the case of a Canadian girl – the daughter of a doctor – who never felt pain. She had bitten the tip off her tongue, suffered third-degree burns after kneeling on a radiator, and experienced countless lacerations in childhood. 'She felt no pain when parts of her body were subjected to strong electric shock, to hot water temperature that usually produce reports of burning pain, or to a prolonged ice-bath,' he reports.

> Equally astonishing was the fact that she showed no changes in blood-pressure, heart-rate, or respiration when these stimuli were presented. Furthermore, she could not remember ever sneezing or coughing, the gag reflex could be elicited only with great difficulty, and corneal reflexes (to protect the eyes) were absent. A variety of other stimuli, such as inserting a stick up through the nostrils, pinching tendons, or injections of histamine under the skin – which are normally considered as forms of torture – also failed to produce pain.

Melzack goes on:

> Miss C. had severe medical problems. She exhibited pathological changes in her knees, hip and spine, and underwent several orthopaedic operations. Her surgeon attributed these changes to the lack of protection to joints usually given by pain sensation. She apparently failed to shift her weight when standing, to turn over in her sleep, or to avoid certain postures, which normally prevent inflammation of joints. Miss C. died at the

age of twenty-nine of massive infections that could not be brought under control. During her last month she complained of discomfort, tenderness and pain in the left hip. The pain was relieved by analgesic tablets. There is little doubt that her inability to feel pain until the final month of her life led to the extensive skin and bone trauma that contributed in a direct fashion to her death.

At the other extreme are people who feel excruciating pain without reason. A gentle touch, a tickle, even a draught of air on the skin can cause them to register agony, and the pain may persist for hours, long after the stimulus has been removed.

Dr W.K. Livingston, in *Pain Mechanism* (Macmillan), cites the case of a 58-year-old married woman who came to him complaining of recurring pain in her right foot. She had fallen three years previously and injured it.

The outer side of the foot [he reports] turned 'black and blue' but X-ray plates did not reveal any fractures. As the ecchymosis [discoloration] cleared she noted that the outer three toes 'felt dead'. Later she began to have periodic pains 'like a toothache' in these toes, and during such attacks all three would be extremely sensitive to touch. The attacks continued with increasing frequency and severity, sometimes occurring several times a day, and occasionally skipping a day or two, but never longer. . . . The subjective feeling of 'deadness' seemed to increase just before an attack began. Next she experienced a sensation of swelling in the toes beginning at their bases on the plantar [sole] surface and spreading to involve all three toes to their junction with the foot. . . . At its height, she said the toes felt 'as if bursting and on fire'. During the attack she was unable to tolerate the lightest touch to the toes. She had never noted any change in colour, temperature or sweating of these toes even during an attack. For the previous two years the outer three toes of the other foot had felt 'slightly numb and dead', and on several occasions she had experienced twinges of pain in them which made her fear that 'the trouble is going over into the other foot'. Nothing of significance was found in physical examination. She received ten injections of a 2 per cent Novocaine solution into the [bottom] of the foot at the base of the toes. Each injection was followed by a period of complete relief from attacks, and these intervals of freedom became increasingly long as the treatment progressed.

Nobody can yet explain such irrational pain. But it sometimes drives its victims repeatedly to seek surgery in an effort to obtain relief, and it has even been known to lead to suicide.

RESISTANCE TO PAIN

These extremes apart, there is evidence that all normal people start with the same basic ability to feel – the same 'threshold' of sensation – in their nervous systems. What alters is their individual concept of pain. As Dr Harold Merskey of the National Hospital, Queen Square, London, puts it:

> Most, if not all, workers consider that thresholds for the complaint of pain depend upon physiological factors which are relatively constant from person to person and group to group.
>
> However, the threshold is usually thought to vary somewhat with sex, occupation, cultural attitudes, ethnic group and mood. Thus women tend to have lower thresholds than men; labourers and miners have higher thresholds than clerical workers; and anxious patients have lower thresholds than those who are not anxious [*Journal of Psychosomatic Research*, vol. 17].

Two American research workers, R. A. Sternback and Dr B. Tursky, investigated sensation threshold in 1964. They gave mild electric shocks to four groups of women – Jews, Italians, Americans and Irish. The women were asked to speak out at the first detectable tingling. All reacted at exactly the same level of stimulus.

Nevertheless, ethnic background *can* have an influence on attitude to pain. This was demonstrated in 1960 by three Canadian research workers – Wallace Lambert, Eva Libman and Ernest Poser – who tried two separate experiments comparing Protestants with Jews. In the first experiment, forty Protestant women and forty Jewish women (all aged 18–23) were asked to allow their arms to be squeezed in an uncomfortable pressure-cuff. A reading was taken at the first moment when pain was felt and another when the pain became intolerable. The cuff was then released and each volunteer was asked to submit to a further test five minutes later, 'to establish reliability'. During the intervening five minutes, half the women in each group were told, casually, that there was scientific evidence that Jews were less willing to endure pain than non-Jews, and that the whole purpose of the experiment was to prove or disprove this. A second set of pain measurements was then taken.

The result was conclusive. Jewesses who had been told of the reputation of Jewry for 'cissiness' raised their pain-acceptance levels markedly. Protestants kept theirs approximately the same.

'We conclude', say the three research workers, 'that the Jewesses were clearly influenced by the interpolated statement which alluded to Jewish "inferiority" with regard to withstanding pain. The fact that an equivalent, provoking statement had no apparent effect on Protestants can be interpreted as meaning that Protestantism does not function as a reference group in the same sense that Judaism does' (*Journal of Personality*, vol. 28).

The second experiment involves eighty Jewesses and eighty Christian women (mostly Catholics). This time, two experimenters were present at each pain-test – 'one recognizably Jewish, the other recognizably non-Jewish'. In the interval between the two pain-tests, thirty of the Jewesses were told that it had been reported in literature that Jews were less able to withstand pain than Christians, and thirty were told the reverse. Similarly, two matching groups of Christians were indoctrinated. The remainder were told nothing.

Once again, the Jews upped their pain-acceptance levels. But this time, so did some of the Christians – those who felt their religious group was under attack. 'Our findings of more homogeneous reactions to pain among Jews would suggest that something like an ideal pattern of reactions to pain is either more standardized and/or more effectively communicated among Jews than Christians,' add the researchers.

I have already referred to the influence which the Crucifixion had on the mental attitudes of Christians towards suffering and pain throughout nineteen centuries. A similar 'grin and bear it' complex was induced in hundreds of thousands of Englishmen in the late nineteenth and early twentieth centuries by the public school system, which ennobled boxing and rugby, and conditioned minds to make light of pain by repeated cold showers, canings and cross-country runs.

Indian fakirs are masters of the art of ignoring pain. I have personally seen a man walk across a pit of hot coals and stones and another lie near-naked on a bed of sharp nails. Neither, so far as one could tell, had taken drugs: they had merely adjusted their mental attitudes. In India also, it is possible to witness 'hook-hanging'. This ancient ceremony is supposed to convey the desire of the gods to bless children and crops. A villager is chosen to represent 'god' and steel hooks are driven into his back. He is then placed on a cart and driven from village to village, suspended from a pole solely by the hooks. The look of entrancement on his face betrays no indication of pain. Yogis in India frequently undergo minor surgery without anaesthetics or pain-killers; they simply concentrate the mind on some distant object or sound and so blot out all other sensations. Attitude of mind is all-important if pain is to be ignored successfully. In 1973, Amnesty International published a *Report on Torture* which stated:

> The best and most commonplace resistance to pain and stress . . . is the simple denial that it is either a potent pain or stress or even a pain or stress at all. This denial may be either culturally or individually generated. For example, the removal of a finger-nail by a surgeon, although uncomfortable, is patiently borne in the knowledge that it will produce relief of pain and a return to normal health . . . [but] the pulling off of a finger-nail under coercive interrogation, or the insertion of needles into the quick, is a horrendous experience and pain is dramatically different from that experienced in the benevolent surgical context.

It seems hard to believe that a 23-year-old woman could resist this kind of torture:

> After a short while, they forced me to take off my skirt and stockings and laid me down and tied my hands and feet to pegs. A person . . . beat the soles of my feet for half an hour. Later they attached wires to my fingers and toes and passed electric current through my body. At the same time they kept beating my naked thighs with truncheons. . . . After a while, they disconnected the wire from my finger and connected it to my ear. They immediately gave it a high dose of electricity. My whole body and head shook in a terrible way. My front teeth started breaking. At the same time, my torturers would hold a mirror to my face and say, 'Look what is happening to your lovely green eyes.'

But resist she did.

Pain can actually come as a relief in the course of some tortures. This is how one Brazilian researcher describes electrical shock to the limbs:

> The tortured victim shouts with all his might, grasping for a footing, somewhere to stand in the midst of that chaos of ·convulsions, shaking and sparks. He cannot lose himself or turn his attention away from that desperate sensation. For him,

in that moment, any other form of combined torture – paddling, for example – would be a relief, for it would allow him to divert his attention, touch ground and his own body which feels like it is escaping his grasp. Pain saves him, beating comes to his rescue. He tries to cause himself pain by beating his head repeatedly on the ground. But generally he is tied, hanging in the 'pau de arara' (parrot's perch), and not even that resource is available to him [Paulo Schilling, *Brasil: seis anos de dictadura y torturas,* 1970].

Amnesty International pointed out that excruciatingly painful procedures, such as electric shocks to the genitalia, can be borne by some prisoners who may then find it impossible to resist the threat to administer a painless 'truth drug'. It all depends on one's attitude of mind. And the mind, when it comes to pain, is capable of some quite extraordinary things.

THE MAN WITHOUT A FACE

Aquila Airways Flight 101 to Lisbon had just taken off from Southampton Water. The sky was clear and moonlit, the sea was smooth, and the sixty-nine passengers aboard began to relax as the flying-boat climbed steadily towards its cruising altitude of 10,000 feet.

Then, an engine spluttered. 'Sounds like magneto trouble,' thought the airline's sales manager, Peter Carey. He felt the flying-boat bank to starboard as if to head back to the Solent. He was sitting with his back to a bulkhead separating the crew from the passenger cabin, and he leaned forward to look out of a porthole.

The next few minutes of that early morning of 15 November 1957 are a blank in Peter Carey's life.

He knew nothing of the crash. He vaguely remembered his head being snapped forward and slammed into his chest by the bulkhead behind. And he has a vivid recollection of coming round to discover himself in the middle of a blazing inferno, with smoke, flames and screams coming from all sides. His clothes were on fire. His hair was singed off. His hands were scorched and stinging. In his own words, he 'felt a draught of air and saw a black patch in the ring of fire – I lunged at it, shouting to the other passengers: "Come this way." '

Believing himself to be several hundred – if not thousand – feet in the air, he prayed as he jumped. 'I thought I was jumping to eternity,' he explained. 'Instead I found myself dropping only about forty feet and then running like hell through a quarry.'

He carried on running until a soldier stopped him and helped to beat out the flames still searing his body. Then he lay still until a doctor injected him with morphine and a helicopter came to take him to the Wessex Regional Burns Unit at Odstock Hospital, Southampton.

And that was the beginning of a painful and quite remarkable fight back to normal life for a man who had become literally faceless. In his own words: 'A few days later I realized that the only bit left of my face was a small area of flesh under the nose, like a Charlie Chaplin moustache: the rest had been burned away. But I was lucky to be alive.'

History shows that the Solent flying-boat had struck the face of a quarry near Newport, Isle of Wight, and had hung like a fly for a few moments – its tail snapped off – before slithering down and disintegrating. In those few moments, Peter Carey had jumped through the hole in the fuselage; he was one of only three survivors.

In the hospital ward he saw many severely burned patients 'give up the ghost'. He nearly did so himself. 'I was lying in bed one morning, feeling incredibly low,' he recalls,

> The pain had been terrible for days. It would have been so easy at that moment to let go and just slip away into death. Then I heard a Cockney voice come through the door and say to the nurse beside my bed: ' 'Ave you 'adya cuppa, dearie?' and it made me laugh. I thought: 'God – what am I doing?' After that, I never had any more problems with myself.

He developed a technique for dealing with pain. 'I made myself believe that the pain was only in one half of my body,' he explained. 'Every morning I would wake up and mentally drive the pain into, say, my left half. I would then think only of my right side. Next day I would drive it across to the right, and think only of my left. I found that, that way, I could live with the pain – it only seemed half as bad.'

Unfortunately, one by one, his features dropped off – nose, ears, eyelids, tops of fingers. But one by one, the surgeons grafted on new ones, or artificial substitutes.

It has taken more than twenty years to rebuild his face, but he has now regained a sort of handsomeness. He has become a successful business executive, managing a chain of travel agents.

'I shall never forget the pain,' he says, 'but perhaps there is a greater scar – the memory of the incredible cruelty of some of my fellow-men. Some people will come up to you in the street and say "If I had a face like yours, I'd shoot myself," or "How dare you come out looking like that." '

DO WOMEN FEEL PAIN MORE THAN MEN?

This particular argument was once put to the test in the radiotherapy department of a London teaching hospital in 1965, when forty-seven patients with tumours were asked to report how bad they felt their pain to be, assessing it on a scale of 0–10. 0 indicated no pain, 10 'as bad as it could possibly be'. A nurse noted what pain-relieving drugs were given.

Male patients rated their pain as more severe. They also asked for relief more often.

But a leading article in *The Lancet* in 1971 stated: 'Thresholds tend to be lower in women than men, in those from lower socio-economic groups and in people engaged in sedentary occupations, compared with those doing hard physical work.'

Not surprisingly, psychologists find there is a relationship between ability to withstand pain and extroversion; in other words, the more of a showman you are, the more pain you are willing to accept without complaining.

The Lancet (June 1971, p.1284) relates:

By means of the extroversion/introversion neuroticism/stability dimensions developed by Eysenck, it has been shown that introverts have lower threshold for pain than extroverts, but the former complain less readily than the latter, who are thought to 'exaggerate' their experiences. Both forms of behaviour have advantages, for introverts, being 'non-complainers', are regarded with favour for their stoicism, whereas extroverts, although 'complainers', usually gain access most readily to analgesics. The idea of 'exaggeration' of complaints arises from the observations of Petrie and others that some individuals process stimuli by reducing them (reducers), some by increasing them (augmenters), whereas others do neither (moderates). Reducers are more than usually tolerant of pain and less of all-round reduction in environment stimulation, whereas augmenters are less tolerant of pain and more of sensory deprivation. Thus, reducers are similar to extroverts and augmenters to introverts. Clearly, there is a difference between tolerance of pain and complaint behaviour.

More detailed information about personality structure and pain has been provided. In a group of women with advanced cancer, stable extroverts were pain-free, and introverts with raised emotionality experienced pain but tended not to complain. Extroverted patients with increased emotionality experienced pain and complained, and together with introverts with increased emotionality, had had more painful or psychologically determined illness in the past than the stable extroverts.

The Lancet adds: 'Information providing a basis for improving our knowledge of pain is thus emerging. The plea for individual assessments of patients' pain, rather than the acceptance of traditional views that disorders of a similar type are equally painful or painless, deserve support.'

Age can have an influence on pain. The slap which makes a child cry will rarely bring tears from an adult. Conversely, some people claim to become more sensitive to pain as old age approaches, possibly because they find themselves with more time to think about it.

PAIN AT NIGHT

The time of day can have an effect on pain. Job complained in the Bible: 'My bones are pierced in me in the night season.' Toothache usually feels worse at night. After a survey of pain at night carried out at the Westminster Hospital in London, three doctors reported:

> It is in the small hours that pain is less bearable. During the night, the unoccupied mind has more time to dwell on the lack of progress in some chronic disorder and on the apparent failure of different forms of therapy. It is then that depression and anxiety mount in all of us. To get through the day is hard enough a fight for the patient with crippling osteo-arthritis or severe rheumatoid arthritis, but when nights have been sleepless and pain-wracked, the next day is started with physical and psychological stores depleted and the patient already exhausted at the starting-post. A number of painful disorders are worse at night and in the early morning [*The Lancet* 25 April 1970, p.881].

They included rheumatoid arthritis, ankylosing spondylitis, degenerative joint disease, gout and tumours of the bone, although for some of these there was a physical explanation for the fluctuations in pain.

The doctors – F. D. Hart, R. T. Taylor and E. C. Huskisson – first investigated cycles of pain in arthritics. They concluded: 'The worst period in the twenty-four hours for the patient with rheumatoid arthritis is usually the waking hours in the early morning. 100 patients attending our clinic were asked which was their worst time of day: 60 said that it was on waking and 16 found the night the worst time; only 22 found the day-time or evening the worst.'

They went on:

Although overuse of diseased joints produces aggravation of symptoms, so does underuse. The morning 'gelling' or fixing of the swollen, inflamed tissues follows a night's rest; a hot bath and a period of exercises are required to dispel this painful stiffness. The 'limbering-up time' is a rough, but useful, measure of clinical progress. In the early morning, swelling of finger and other joints is maximal and the grip strength minimal.

Patients with ankylosing spondylitis, they found, were usually in most pain at night or early morning:

The patient wakes stiff and painful, and may take three or four hours to become sufficiently mobile to dress and go to work. One patient sets his alarm clock at two to three hourly intervals throughout the night, otherwise morning stiffness does not allow him to commute to the office where he works. Another rises from his bed painfully stiff at about 3.30 a.m., exercises, smokes a cigarette, then props himself up sitting on the floor with his back hard against the wall, and there remains for the rest of the night.

Of gout they had this to say: 'Gout is the classic example of nocturnal agony. Attacks characteristically start in the small hours, and therapy started immediately, as soon as the pain has awoken the patient, is more productive of rapid relief than when it is delayed some hours.'

'For some patients with metastatic bone disease,' they added, 'there is no ease by day or night, in or out of bed. Such patients are often found in hospital painfully walking the corridors during the night, afraid of returning to bed for fear of an exacerbation of their pain.'

PAIN IN THE BONES

There is a saying 'I can feel it in my bones.' Some people claim that they can feel pain actually 'in their bones'. But can they?

Bone is a hard substance. It is difficult, therefore, to slice or chop into sections for examination under the microscope. Furthermore, if you soften it first – by removing some of the calcium – you alter the nature of the material inside and so ruin it for scientific investigation.

To this day, no medical research has been able to detect the existence of nerves in bone on a microscope slide, and so most medical authorities doubt that it is possible to feel pain 'in the bones'. Every bone is sheathed – rather like the handle of a cricket bat – with a flexible membrane known as the periosteum. The periosteum contains masses of nerves and until recently it was thought to be this – and this alone – which conveyed pain if a bone was damaged or broken. But Ralph Denham, consultant orthopaedic surgeon to the Royal Portsmouth Hospital, had doubts. . . .

At 6 p.m. on a grey, mid-March evening in 1972, a team of orthopaedic surgeons had just completed a strenuous operation to equip a patient with an artificial hip. During the operation, Ralph Denham – the senior surgeon present – had become a little worried. On the palm of his right hand, a small cyst – a *Dupuytrenes nodule* – had appeared and was causing him some discomfort.

'I think', he told his colleagues, 'I'm going to have to take a few days off and have this attended to.'

Next morning, he had an idea. For some months, he had been trying to find an explanation for the fact that about one in ten of the hip replacement operations which he performed ended in failure, with the patient feeling intense pain whenever he put weight on to the newly-installed, artificial hip. Why?

Denham put forward a plan to his colleagues. 'I have a strong suspicion', he told his team at Portsmouth, 'that the pain which these patients feel comes from within the bone itself. I know it sounds silly, but I want to try a little experiment.'

At 4 p.m. that day he climbed on to a trolley and had himself wheeled into the operating theatre. He persuaded his colleagues to give him a general anaesthetic and to cut open both his legs, so as to expose the shin-bone (tibia). Before losing consciousness, he requested that they strip back the periosteum on one – to the extent of about six inches – but not on the other.

Finally, he handed them four stainless-steel screws. The screws were two inches long (I have one on the desk in front of me as I write). Two were inserted into one leg, two into the other. The assisting surgeon first drilled four holes: two completely through the the shin-bones, the other two half-way through. A screw was placed in each hole and tightened. Finally, dressings were placed on the wounds so that only the heads of the screws poked through.

When Ralph Denham came round, it was impossible to tell which screw was which. Nor did he know from which of his legs the periosteum membrane – with its supply of nerves – had been stripped. He slept satisfied. Next morning, one of his colleagues appeared with a screwdriver. Half a turn at a time, he tightened each screw.

'The result of the experiment', Ralph Denham records:

> . . . was absolutely identical on both sides – the stripped side
> was as painful as the unstripped side. When the half-inserted
> screw touched the far cortex (outer layer) of bone in each leg, it
> really did hurt quite a lot. Furthermore, when my colleague
> slowed down to a quarter-turn at a time – because I was
> grumbling a bit – I could identify quite positively which screw
> had gone right through the bone and which had gone only part
> of the way through. The ones which had gone all the way
> through were only slightly uncomfortable, whereas the ones
> which began to touch the cortex as he screwed them in were
> really awfully sore. Another interesting thing – the pain
> would die away after each quarter-turn, within a minute or so.
> But with each fresh turn, the pain would come back. It was like
> a thumb-screw in a torture chamber.

The surgeon's final observation was that removal of the screws was
as painful as having them screwed in: 'It seems that the *rate of change*
of the stimulus governs the degree of pain felt,' he added, 'which fits
in with the laws of pain for other parts of the body.'

Despite his own personal discomfort – 'I had to forgo my usual
skiing holiday for one year' – Ralph Denham was delighted. He had
certainly proved, at least to his own satisfaction, that you *could* feel
pain in bones. And he immediately put the lesson into practice.

Until then, the operation to fit an artificial hip at the Royal
Portsmouth Hospital had been of the type known to orthopaedic
surgeons as 'the Ring operation'. During it, a plastic socket (*cup*) is
attached to the pelvis and a stainless steel spike (with a ball on the
end, to fit into the socket) is driven down into the thigh-bone. A
flange on the spike prevents it going too far by coming into contact
with a ring of bone. What Ralph Denham had begun to suspect was
that sometimes the flange failed to settle properly on to the ring of
bone, and that when the patient started to walk and put weight on it
the pressure of the spike inside caused the bone to swell. Such
swelling could well be the cause of the pain – if, that is, bones had
nerves inside them which could transmit pain.

> Imagine the thigh-bone as a tube and the femoral component
> of the artificial hip (the spiky part) as a triangular wedge
> pressing down into that tube. . . . As the patient walks, so the
> wedge – if it is at all loose – forces the tube to dilate. We know
> that elsewhere in the body, tubes don't like being made to

dilate – if you eat green apples you get painful colic, and so forth – and it may be that bones react in the same way.

He decided to modify the operation. Instead of forcing the spiked section of the artificial hip straight down into the thigh-bone, he filled the cavities in the bone first with a special cement (a technique pioneered by John Charnley, consultant orthopaedic surgeon to the Wrighton Hospital, Lancashire). The acrylic cement set within ten minutes, holding the stainless steel spike rock-firm. No wobble, no pain.

Today, Ralph Denham likes to think of nerves in bones as tendrils of ivy entwined around the marble columns of a temple.

'Bones are up-and-down structures,' he explains:

> They are arranged inside rather like marble columns – called osteones – and when you break a bone you break the columns. It seems to me that if you were the Lord and you were trying to organize a protective mechanism for bones, you would arrange for something like ivy (nerves) to weave a way between the columns so that if the tendrils felt the rumblings of an earthquake they could somehow effect a buttressing-up operation. Obviously, they would have to accept the normal weight of the roof of the temple without reacting, otherwise they would shout at you every time you stood up: any nerves in bones should only fire off in the presence of an *ab*normal stimulus, not in the presence of a normal one.

THE LANGUAGE OF PAIN

Some doctors have been known to classify pain under three different headings: 'pricking', 'burning' or 'aching'. But the ancient Arab physician Abu-Ali Avicenna preferred fifteen. And in 1970, Professor Ronald Melzack and his Canadian colleague, W. S. Torgerson, scoured medical literature and came up with 102 adjectives used to describe pain.

They divided them into three main classes: 'sensory' (words which describe the duration, area, pressure or heat of pain), 'affective' (describing tension or fear) and 'evaluative' (describing, from the patient's point of view, the over-all intensity of the pain). They sub-divided them into thirteen sub-classes.

They then gave the list of words – broken down into their classes – to twenty-eight men and twelve women (all university students or graduates) and asked them whether they agreed that the words correctly described pain. They found a very high measure of agreement, as the following table shows:

CLASS	WORD	PERCENTAGE AGREEMENT
Temporal (around the temples)	Pounding, Pulsing, Throbbing	100%
	Thumping	95%
	Beating	90%
	Flickering, Quivering	70%
Spatial (describing spread)	Shooting	90%
	Spreading, Darting, Radiating	85%
	Flashing	75%
	Jumping	65%
Punctuate pressure (caused by a point)	Stabbing, Piercing	100%
	Penetrating	85%
	Drilling, Lancinating, Pricking	75%
	Boring	70%
Incisive pressure (caused by a sharp edge)	Cutting	95%
	Sharp	80%
	Lacerating	65%
	Tearing	55%
Constrictive pressure (encircling pressure)	Cramping	100%
	Crushing, Pressing, Squeezing	95%
	Binding, Gripping	85%
	Pinching	80%
	Nipping	70%
	Biting, Gnawing, Tight	65%
	Taut	50%
Traction pressure	Pulling, Tugging	90%
	Wrenching	85%
	Grinding	30%
Thermal	Burning	100%
	Scalding	90%
	Searing, Hot	80%
Brightness	Smarting, Tingling	90%
	Stinging	85%
	Tickling	80%
	Rasping, Itchy	55%

CLASS	WORD	PERCENTAGE AGREEMENT
Dullness	Aching, Blurred, Dull, Numbing	95%
	Heavy	80%
	Sore, Steady	75%
	Drawing, Hurting	65%
	Tender	60%
	Blinding	25%
	Splitting	20%
Tension	Fatiguing, Tiring	100%
	Exhausting, Dragging	90%
	Nagging	70%
Autonomic	Sickening, Nauseating	95%
	Suffocating	90%
	Choking	85%
	Wretched	40%
Fear	Terrifying, Frightful	95%
	Fearful	85%
	Dreadful	75%
	Awful	30%
Punishment	Gruelling, Killing, Torturing	95%
	Punishing, Racking, Vicious	85%
	Cruel	65%
	Wicked	60%
Evaluating	Annoying, Horrible, Intolerable	95%
	Agonizing, Mild, Troublesome, Miserable, Unbearable	90%
	Bearable, Distressing, Intense	85%
	Discomforting, Distracting	80%
	Violent, Excruciating	75%
	Savage	70%
	Ugly	65%

Which words, then, should be used to describe which types of pain? There is no absolute agreement, no standard. But, broadly speaking, pain caused by inflammation can usually be called 'throbbing'; pain in bones may be 'excruciating' or 'penetrating'; pain due to a growth is probably 'gnawing'; overaction of a muscle or a weak part may produce 'aching'; excess acid in the stomach leads to a 'burning' sensation; and colic – or any other inflammation of internal ducts – is perhaps best described as 'griping'.

Beyond these broad categories, it is very much a matter of how vocal, observant or educated the patient is and how much his doctor is prepared to press him. As Virginia Woolf says in her essay 'On Being Ill', 'English, which can commonly express the thoughts of Hamlet and the tragedy of Lear, has no words for the shiver and the headache. . . . The merest schoolgirl, when she falls in love, has Shakespeare and Keats to speak for her; but let a sufferer try to describe a pain in his head to a doctor and language at once runs dry.'

Melzack and Torgerson say they are now trying to devise a questionnaire which could be used to help determine the nature and course of pain. But they add a word of warning: 'The fact that there are so many words to describe the experience of pain lends support to the concept that the word 'pain' is a label which represents a myriad of different experiences, and refutes the traditional concept that pain is a single modality which carries one or two qualities.'

PAIN IN HOSPITAL

To try to throw more light on people's attitudes to pain, I asked a research worker at Charing Cross Hospital, Ruth Levitt, if she would be willing to discuss pain with patients during the course of her normal rounds. The hospital management kindly gave permission, and so Ruth drew up a questionnaire which included such questions as 'What sort of pain do you have?', 'Can you get relief from it?', 'What do you feel about telling a nurse you are in pain?', 'Are some doctors whom you have seen easier to talk to about the pain than others?', 'Is it different talking to someone here about your pain, compared with telling a friend or someone in your family?', 'When another patient talks to you about his or her pain, what do you feel?' and 'What is the worst kind of pain you have ever had?'

Ruth found an extraordinary reluctance on the part of most of the hospital patients to talk about their pain. She says in her report to me:

1. The patients I spoke to found it difficult to put their own private experience of pain into words which adequately described what they felt. This was because, in the hospital

environment, they were accustomed only to reporting on the intensity of their pain and whether or not it was getting better. They were not used to finding words and images to convey the quality of the sensations they felt.

2. They said they were not reticent about reporting their pain to doctors and nurses provided that (a) they were asked to do so, and (b) the pain was 'bad enough' to warrant reporting. They did not talk to other patients specifically about their pain – 'everyone has enough of their own troubles' – although they might mention it in passing (if they had conversations about why they had had to come into hospital). Talking to close family about pain was more complicated because it evoked anxiety and sympathy from them – responses with which it might be difficult to cope: at least with doctors and nurses it was 'their job' to hear reports of pain from patients.

3. Some patients were upset or alarmed by seeing other patients in pain or hearing them talk about it. Most patients said they were not unduly affected by this. Most felt that it was really up to each individual patient to see that he got enough relief and did not have to suffer excessively. The patients I spoke to said that they were not particularly concerned if people at work or at home reported pain, for similar reasons, although most agreed that if a child reported pain (provided they were convinced that it was genuine) they would feel more concerned and sympathetic, since children were less able to cope with pain than adults.

With one exception, my impression was that the words patients used did not really do justice to the depth and variety of their experience, and that there were powerful social constraints preventing them from 'letting themselves go'. These constraints could be a function both of the individual's own upbringing, and of the social environment created in the hospital.

Some patients clearly thought that they would appear childish, and might be ridiculed or humiliated, if they admitted to distress or anguish as a result of being in pain. Some felt it was their duty as patients to be bright and cheerful, so that other patients and staff would not be burdened by their private anxieties and problems.

And the exception?

He was a boy of nineteen who had been suffering from severe kidney disease since he was four years old. He was about to receive a donated kidney in a transplantation operation, the new kidney being donated by his younger brother. He first described the 'numb' pain in his ankle following insertion of a 'shunt', before the transplantation could proceed. Then he remembered a pain that had been much worse. It was when he had had a bone biopsy, the slice being taken from his femur under local anaesthetic. He said it was very distressing because the anaesthetic did not block all sensation from the site and he had felt the needle being inserted and scraping inside the bone. When the effect of the anaesthetic had worn off, the combination of sharp and dull pain in his thigh was very hard to bear.

Then he remembered that, really, the worse pain he had ever had was from the severe headaches which he suffered when his blood-pressure went up. It had seemed to be quite impossible to reduce the intensity, either with drugs or by trying to think about something else. He said that when he was younger he had suffered all sorts of pains and had never said anything about it to his parents or anyone else because he did not understand what the pains were nor why *he* should have them. In the last two years, after frequent spells in hospital, he had learned how seriously ill he was and now did not hesitate to report if he was in pain, because he realized it was doing him no good to go on suffering. He also realized that it was important to tell doctors and nurses the details of how he felt. He said he would only tell another person about his own pain if it would help that person with theirs. He cited as an example the time when, following his decision to be a donor, his brother had had to have an intravenous pyelogram (this involves injection of a radio-opaque dye followed by a series of X-rays to demonstrate the kidney's structure and functioning). The boy himself had undergone this procedure before and knew that, when the dye is injected, you suddenly feel a hot burning pain all through the body. So, he told his brother about it beforehand. His brother told him afterwards that, without the warning, he would have feared – as a result of the sudden pain – that he was about to die.

Ruth Levitt was only able to put her questions to eight patients – and have longer interviews with three more – before she had to resume her other work. She concludes:

The number of patients used in this project was not large enough to regard their views as being statistically representative. Nevertheless, the results suggest that there is a great deal of important material waiting to be tapped, but that this requires a more sophisticated technique – one which can by-pass the strong, social taboos that can restrain people from discussing pain more fully. 'Social taboos' may include not wishing to appear ungrateful or fear of upsetting the ministering angel. I am absolutely convinced – from personal observation – that the treatment of pain in hospital is handled far too often as a *routine*, rather than as a specific prescription to suit the individual patient. The drugs trolley always seems to take the same route around the ward, regardless of whether the person in the last bed may be in greater pain than anyone else that day. The drugs to be issued are rarely discussed with the patient.

In a letter to *The Lancet* in 1971, Dr James Parkhouse of Manchester University's Department of Anaesthetics, wrote: 'The truth is, obviously enough, that the routine prescribing of standard doses of analgesics can never be an ideal way of catering for individual patients. What can be said of it is that it can be done without making great demands on the time and skill of health personnel.' Dr Parkhouse goes on:

There is still a tendency to think in averages, to assume that because simple mastectomy is not generally a painful procedure the occasional patient who complains bitterly must be, so to speak, a liar or a fool. Thus, severe pain and discomfort sometimes do, regrettably, pass unheeded. There is also the other side of the story: I well remember anaesthetizing a young woman for a simple operation on the groin, an hour or two after which she was sitting up contentedly in bed with no complaint of pain. When I saw her the following morning – pale, nauseated, and dizzy – she was scarcely recognizable as the same person. She complained with tears in her eyes that she would be perfectly all right if only she didn't have to have the injections, which turned out to be the 'routine' post-operative 'Omnopon'.

I would, however, enter a further plea for the employment of trained nurses, attached to departments of anaesthetics and surgery, with the primary responsibility for attending to the patient's comfort. This work can effectively and humanely be combined, as has been said before, with the controlled clinical evaluation of analgesics. In employing nurses in this way over a number of years it has been my experience, and that of others, that when fear and anxiety have been replaced by encouragement and understanding, and when the many sources of discomfort in the post-operative period have been sought and put right, the need for powerful analgesics is not as universal as might be supposed. They can then, as is proper, be given to the right patients, at the right times, and in the right doses.

Dr Harold Merskey, in an article in the *Nursing Times* in August 1971, admitted:

> Doctors and nurses do not always have a good reputation among patients for their efforts to relieve pain. Frequently one hears of patients whom the staff thinks 'complain too much' about their pain. And patients, perhaps relieved of some illness which endangered life, have been known to bitterly criticize the staff who saved them, because too little thought was given to caring for their distress in the process of their cure. Before we decide that too many patients are simply ungrateful, it is worth considering why this happens.
>
> One reason, of course, is that nurses and doctors – but perhaps especially doctors – approach symptoms from very different angles compared with the patient. Apart from the fact that doctors and nurses do not usually, one hopes, have the symptoms which distress patients, their aim is firstly to make a diagnosis and only later to relieve the presenting symptoms. The patient is much less interested in diagnosis and its refinements – he wants to be free from his discomfort first and only secondly might he be interested to know what it was that went wrong.

Dr Merskey goes on:

> It is true that from the doctor's point of view all will be satisfactory once the problems of diagnosis and appropriate treatment have been solved (although this may not mean recovery for the hapless patient). But what the patient wants is relief from his pain, and from the attendant anxiety which pain and illness nearly always bring. Too often this is neglected or not given sufficient attention.
>
> In theory, nurses make the same error less than doctors since they more often take up their profession in order to provide treatment and comfort than do doctors. However, in fact, nurses too are quite likely to fall into the same trap as their

medical colleagues, and this naturally happens most readily in highly sophisticated units where nurses take over some of the technical work and attitudes of the doctor, like blood-pressure recording, machine monitoring, collection of numerous samples and so forth.

Finally, he adds: 'A less obvious but more fundamental reason is that doctors and nurses tend to forget what pain is all about. . . .'

THE VALUE OF PAIN

'Nature's warning', 'the cry of an injured nerve', 'a speedometer of damage' – these are some of the descriptions which have been given to the function of pain. And it is true that, more often than not, it serves a useful purpose.

If you tread on a nail, pain helps to speed up the reflex action which withdraws the foot. If you develop an inflammation or a blister, the pain usually enforces rest of the affected part and so speeds recovery. If you have a particular form of heart disease, the pain known as *angina pectoris* may warn you that a build-up of metabolites has occurred in your heart muscle and that you are dangerously close to overloading it. If you eat unripe fruit, the pain of colic may serve as a reminder not to do so again.

Pain can be valuable as an aid to diagnosis too. 'Where does it hurt?' is often the doctor's first question – and for this reason, administration of a pain-killer (which may confuse the patient) is frequently delayed until the diagnosis has been completed. This may help to explain Dr Merskey's remark: 'Doctors and nurses tend to forget what pain is all about.'

I once asked a group of freshly-qualified doctors, which – if a patient complained of being in pain – would be their first reaction: 'What can I give to stop the pain?' or 'I wonder what is causing the pain?' To a man – and woman – they answered: 'I wonder what is causing the pain?'

But if some doctors consider pain too much as an aid to diagnosis – and forget, temporarily, what it is doing to the patient – there is increasing recognition of the need to treat pain in special ways in certain situations. Several hospitals in Britain have now set up 'pain clinics'. These are used especially in the treatment of intractable (stubborn) pain – often associated with malignant disease, neuralgia, vascular problems or bone damage. More will be said about these clinics later: suffice to say, for the present, that the success achieved with them to date suggests that every region in the country ought to have one.

Whilst pain can be of value, it can also be useless in excess. Do we really need to feel the intense pain of, say, rheumatism, cancer, migraine or some of the bone disorders to register the fact that there is something wrong inside us? In the olden days, pain was looked on as a punishment (the Romans called it 'pena', which actually *was* the same word as 'punishment') and it is not surprising that many considered it thus, for frequently it has no other rationale.

Dr Cicely Saunders, who operates a Pain Clinic at St Christopher's Hospice at Penge, in south-east London, observes that terminal pain – the kind of pain experienced during advanced stages of cancer – 'unlike many forms of acute pain, has no useful function':

> Typically this is a constant pain with or without exacerbations. It frequently disturbs the patients at night, and although it is often helped at first by mild analgesics the story they give is of less and less relief lasting for shorter and shorter periods. Its treatment may be summed up under three headings: listening, attention to detail, and skill and confidence in handling analgesics and other drugs.
>
> When it occurs, it adds to the deteriorating illness something which is really an illness in itself – one that has to be considered and treated as such. One of its characteristics is that it gives to patients a sense of isolation and despair so that their mental state may demand as much concern as physical symptoms. For example, they speak, over and over again, of the need for 'attention', and frequently express feelings of rejection.

Such pain can have no value. It must surely appear to the patient as savage punishment, prompting the question 'Why me?' And it is one of the few kinds of pain over which the mind seems to have little control.

THE PROBLEM OF MEASURING PAIN

Pain is a highly subjective experience. One of the problems in attempting to conquer it is measuring it in the first place. Sometimes humans are not the best subjects for experiment.

As Dr Gary Blane, a pharmacologist formerly with Reckitt & Colman, explains:

> The results you get when you deliberately inflict pain on humans in the laboratory do not always correlate with what you get with pathological pain, because of the tremendous psychological overtones. If I say to someone: 'Look, I'm going

to put this soldering iron on your foot: relax, there's nothing to worry about, you'll be all right, then – as has happened in the case of one or two volunteers – I can practically burn a hole in their foot before they say 'Ouch – that hurts!' It's a very different thing when you wake up one morning and suddenly feel a little pain in your breast: a very low level of pain will make you say 'Gosh, I must see a doctor straightaway.'

Because of these 'psychological overtones', scientists wishing to test the effectiveness of pain-killing drugs have to make many of their initial measurements on animals. There is a better chance, with an animal, of getting an accurate reaction. Experiments are carried out in accordance with a strict code of practice laid down by the Home Office, and they fall into four main types: pinching, pressing, stimulating by electrical shock and heating.

A typical 'pinching' experiment would be to place an artery clip on a mouse's tail and count how many seconds elapse before it turns round and tries to bite the clip. The time taken under the influence of various pain-killing drugs would be a measure of the analgesic properties of those drugs.

A typical 'pressing' experiment would be to use a special syringe on a dog's paw. Instead of the normal needle, the syringe has a wedge of perspex: mounted on top of the plunger is a pressure-gauge. The researcher places the wedge on the dog's paw and notes how much air-pressure builds up in the barrel of the syringe before the dog complains. Under normal conditions, 5 lb per square inch might be sufficient to produce a bark: after administration of a pain-killer, it might take 20 lb.

A typical 'stimulation' experiment would be to run an electric current through the wire grid on which a rat is living and see how quickly it leaps on to an insulated pole; or embed wires into a tooth of a dog and 'stimulate' the tooth.

A typical 'heating' experiment would be to blacken the tail of a rat and then focus a beam of heat on to it to see how many seconds elapse before it flicks its tail out of the way; or dip the tail into hot water.

Researchers agree that it is usually possible to extrapolate from these experiments on animals the responses to pain in humans. Nevertheless, when it comes to the final stages of the development of a pain-killer, human behaviour must be studied directly. For this purpose, a variety of pain-measuring instruments have been developed for use on volunteers, including one at the Royal College of Surgeons in London called an 'analgesiometer'. 'We simply burn forearms,' explained Professor Jimmy Payne, director of the

Anaesthetics Research Department at the Royal College, waving a hand in the direction of a wedge-shaped metal box on the laboratory bench, from which a thin beam of light was shining.

The analgesiometer is simply a device for measuring people's reactions to pain, a task anything but simple. Basically, as my friend Paul Vaughan remarked when he first saw it, 'It reminds one of the trick every schoolboy knows – hold a magnifying glass at the right angle and you can focus the sun's beam on the back of the neck of the boy in front, with satisfying results'.

It consists of a 500-watt bulb in a tin box whose beam is focused on to a perspex cradle in which the 'victim' rests his forearm. A thyristor (electric control) governs the heat from the bulb, which has a 5-centimetre focal length condensor-lens to concentrate the beam on to a spot only one centimetre in diameter.

The 'victim' controls the dose of heat he gets by pushing a button. He pushes it to switch on the beam; he pushes it again as soon as he feels pain; and he pushes it a third time when the pain becomes unbearable. An electric clock counts the seconds between each push and each cry of 'Now!' Using this device, Professor Payne and his colleagues have been able to confirm that the pain 'sensitivity' of most people is the same: they report being able to feel discomfort from the beam after about ten seconds. But their tolerance of pain varies tremendously. 'Some are terrified of being burned and push the button quickly,' he explained, 'others like to appear as heroes.'

One interesting finding is that when under the influence of certain pain-killing drugs (morphine, for example), the subjects will cry 'Now!' but not always push the button: 'It is as though the *nature* of the pain has changed, rather than its intensity.'

A variation on the analgesiometer has been developed at the Royal Infirmary, Glasgow. It is called a 'thermal probe' and consists of a heat source, a temperature controller (adjustable from 30–80 degrees centigrade) and a probe like a soldering iron which can be placed on any part of the patient's body. It costs about £25 to make and weighs about 11 lb. Its inventors, R. J. Mills and Stewart Renfrew, give this description of how it is used:

> In use the probe is heated to a temperature above the pain threshold, which on average takes place in one minute. The power is then switched off and the probe is allowed to cool. At an ambient temperature of 20°C. the rate of cooling is such that the temperature of the probe falls from 70°C. to 45°C. in three minutes. During the cooling period the probe is applied to the skin for two seconds at 2°C. temperature intervals until a temperature is reached where the subject no longer detects a painful stimulus. Normally this temperature lies in

the range 45–55°C. The time taken to measure the pain threshold is approximately three minutes. In practice it is also possible to set the heat control to provide a known constant temperature at the probe in order to compare the effect of a fixed stimulus on different areas of body-surface [*The Lancet*, 10 April 1971].

Another instrument is the 'dolorimeter', or pain thermometer, invented by Dr James Hardy of the University of Pennsylvania and Dr Harold Wolff of Cornell University. Each degree of pain is registered in 'dols'. A pin-prick or some other barely perceptible pain is half a 'dol'; a headache usually registers 2 or 3 'dols'; something extremely painful – like passing a kidney-stone – may top 10 'dols'.

With the aid of this instrument they may have drawn up a 'Severity Chart' for pain which looks like this:

Pain chart

The chart shows the severity of various types of pain. It is based on the results of tests with a pain-measuring dolorimeter. A dol is a unit of measurement on the machine.

DOLS

0-2	Most skin abrasions.
	Most toothaches.
	Many post-operative wounds.
	Most cancer pains.
	Most backaches.
	Arthritis.
	Most neuralgias.
	Nearly all abdominal pain.
	Sinus pains.
2-5	Most migraine headaches.
	Many abdominal pains.
	Many heart attacks.
	Some cancer pains.
	Some backaches.
	Some neuralgias.
5½	*Average person seldom gets beyond here throughout his or her life.*
6-9	Some heart attacks.
	Some burns.
	Some short-lived muscle cramps.

DOLS
6-9   Occasional migraine headaches.
            Some headaches from haemorrhages, infections and
            tumours inside the head.

9-10½   Some labour pains during childbirth.
            Momentary pains from sudden injury.
            Passing of some kidney-stones.
            A burning cigarette held against the skin.

A much simpler chart has been devised by Dr Edward Huskisson
at St Bartholomew's Hospital, London. It consists of a straight,
vertical line with a mark at the bottom and a mark at the top: the
bottom mark represents 'No pain', the top 'Unbearable'.

'I simply ask the patient to point to where, up the line, his pain has
reached,' he explains.

Such charts are interesting as a guide, but they take no account of the
power of some individuals to deny pain – or adjust their sensitivity to
it – should they wish. There are certain psychological disorders in
which pain is actually craved by the individual and severity is a
measure of pleasure. Some masochists, for example, enjoy being
whipped (the usual explanation for this is that, sub-consciously, they
regard themselves as worthless, or guilty of some fault, and wish to
be punished). And I well remember the case of a prostitute suffering
from 'Munchausen's syndrome' (named after Baron Munchausen,
the celebrated fictional liar) who so delighted in showing off the scars
of surgery that she went from hospital to hospital faking symptoms
of agony in an attempt to 'win' exploratory operations. Her
psychiatrist told me he had counted thirty-two cuts on her body.

Other people fake pain merely to elicit sympathy or draw attention to themselves.

PAIN IN SPORT

An interesting insight into the differing mental attitudes of
sportsmen to pain emerge from two interviews which I conducted
for the medical cassette service, 'Auditorium', in 1974 – one with Dr
Stuart Carne, medical adviser to Queens Park Rangers Football
Club, the other with Dr Leon Walkden, medical adviser to the
Rugby Football Union.

'To what extent', I asked Dr Carne, 'do soccer players sham and to
what extent are their injuries genuine?'

'I think the pain is genuine,' he replied,

. . . it is the *interpretation* of the pain which isn't genuine. After all, there's a great ritual about what is to happen when a player falls down. The trainer comes on to the pitch with his sponge, the game is stopped and everyone stands around. It also has a tactical advantage: it slows the game down and gives everyone else a breather. The pain may be quite serious but I am intrigued by the fact that in rugby this doesn't happen.

Dr Walkden gave this explanation:

Rugby is a game for enjoyment. Rugby players are gregarious people and they want, therefore, to share in the game and in the pleasure afterwards. Professional soccer, on the other hand, is not a sport – at least, not if one uses the definition of sport as 'a division from normal occupation'. Therefore, when a soccer player is involved in an injury, his occupation is at risk: for a few seconds his injury is intensely painful and he reacts subconsciously, by expressing anxiety.

Dr Walkden went on: 'Within a few seconds, however, he realizes that there is no unduly severe lesion occurring. But he then has to carry on with the sporting charade: the dressing-room attendant comes on, two minutes respite follows and then – to the applause of the spectators – he gets up and rapidly resumes the game at a gallop.'
Dr Walkden added:

The rugby player has less tension in his life and so avoids the implications of his injury, accepting pain without functional overtones. He will be relieved by the mild nature of his injury, his fellow players will not express too much relief and so, one might say, in a depth of emotional reserve he takes his injury philosophically, gets to his feet and carries on.

I have tried very hard to persuade all-in wrestlers to admit that much of their apparent pain is pure exhibitionism, but they have a binding loyalty to their profession. The nearest that one well-known wrestler – 'quote me and I'll sue you' – came to an admission was this: 'We do get hurt. But the times when we are in pain are not usually the same times as when we make a fuss: when you are being hurt, you're usually too busy trying to get out of the hold to bother about thumping the canvas.'

THE WORST PAIN?

What, then, is the 'worst' pain a person may have to endure? It all depends on experience. As Professor C. A. Keele of the Middlesex Hospital points out: 'Strictly speaking, one can only be sure of one's own experience of pain: the occurrence of pain in others, and in animals, is an inference.'

Perhaps that may explain the expression of Miss A. M. of Newcastle-upon-Tyne, who sought help from her (male) GP for what, to her, was 'the worst pain ever': dysmenorrhea.

The pain always seemed to wake me up at about 3 o'clock in the morning – it always seems to catch you when you are at your lowest. It was a dull, burning sensation in the pit of the stomach. I used to shoot out of bed and go and sit on the lavatory. The burning sensation would come in waves. When it got very bad I used to feel as though I would pass out. I did black out sometimes but not actually faint. I used to get flashes in front of the eyes, ringing bells in the ears, and hot and cold sweats with very bad diarrhoea at the same time, and sometimes I was violently sick. The blood flow would then start. It felt a bit like burning coals trying to get out of the bottom of your stomach. . . .

The pains started about a year after my periods started. I never had regular periods, they always tended to be late. I could never anticipate when they would come – there was sometimes ten days difference – but it struck me that the later they were, the worse the pains were.

After about five hours on the lav. I would be totally flaked out, and go back to bed exhausted and sleep for three or four hours. Then the pains would wake me up again. Then it would be time to go to school.

We were all a bit thrown at home – my mum had never had any trouble like this. We tried all the usual folk remedies – like gin and cocoa – but it obviously wasn't going to get any better so in the end I was sent to the doc.

He wasn't very interested at all. He was a Catholic and I'm sure he thought the whole thing was some sort of obscure punishment for being a woman anyway, and that it was all between me and God. He said that I would grow out of it and patted me on the head and gave me some little white pills, saying 'Take these two days before your period.' I had explained to him that I had no idea when my periods were going to start, so that bit of treatment was next to useless.

I went to other doctors. I would start telling them the symptoms and suddenly I would see a glazed look come over their eyes, fifteen seconds in. I could see the thought going through their minds, 'Oh God – hysterical woman – she's laying it on a bit. Perhaps she wants to be off school or something,' and I would falter and dry up half-way through because I felt they weren't believing a word I said.

The first sympathetic treatment I got was from a woman doctor at university who was on the student-health body. We tried several mild pain-killers which didn't work, but she did say 'Come back if they don't work,' which was marvellous after about six years of trying to get some help.

Finally, we found a hormonal pill which worked. It was terrific. I suddenly realized one day that the damned thing [period] had arrived and I hadn't felt it coming. It was a most amazing thing, and I went rushing back to her shouting 'It's worked, it's worked!'

Unfortunately, when I left university and went back home again, I had to start once more with the male doctors. One of them actually told me to take Epsom salts and walk three bus-stops every day for a week before my period was due!

In the end, I went on to the contraceptive pill and this not only prevented the pain but also regularized the periods. They've been painless ever since.

Dysmenorrhea may have physical causes (for example an under-developed womb, displacement of the womb, clotting menstrual blood, hormonal imbalance or glandular defects) but it can also be brought on, or exacerbated by, psychological factors, such as a feeling of being 'unclean' during the monthly period or that menstruation is the 'curse of woman'.

To what extent Miss A. M.'s experience is typical, only doctors, patients and their parents know. It is not easy for someone who is disbarred from feeling a particular pain on account of their sex, to imagine its severity.

PAIN IN CHILDBIRTH

Many women in Western society regard childbirth as perhaps the worst pain they could suffer. This may be due to a heightened sense of danger – fear for their own survival – or to a refusal to believe that something as large as a baby could pass easily through something as narrow as the vagina. A different attitude to the pain of childbirth is taken in more primitive societies.

The word 'couvade' is derived from the French word 'couver', meaning 'to hatch'. Couvade is still practised in remote parts of South America today. It is the practice of transferring the pain of childbirth from the wife to the husband by suggestion.

Literary references to couvade suggest that it was first practised in Corsica during the first century AD. Wives who became pregnant were encouraged to go on working in the fields until the final stages of labour. As soon as the first labour pain was felt, the husband retired to bed. He would moan and jerk, just as if it were *he* who was having the baby. After the birth he would take the baby in his arms and stay in bed to recover, while his wife returned to work – often the same day.

Sir Henry Head, the neurologist, once wrote in the *British Medical Journal*: 'The mental state of the patient has a notoriously profound influence over the pains originating in the pelvic viscera.' This view is supported by midwives to whom I have spoken, all of whom agree that most severe labour pains are usually felt by (or bemoaned by) women with marital or other emotional problems, or by those who did not wish to become pregnant in the first place.

Dr Grantly Dick-Read, prime advocate of 'natural' (no anaesthetic) childbirth, suggests in his book *Revelation of Childbirth* (Heinemann Medical) that pain only occurs in labour when the mind is unprepared for certain sensations coming from the uterus. Natural contractions of the uterus, he asserts, are misinterpreted by the thalamus in the brain as pain signals. The thalamus then instructs a muscular defence mechanism to leap into action, leading to spasms which cause real pain.

Therefore [he goes on], uterine contractions become painful, and we find that through the misinterpretation of non-injurious stimuli, a painless natural function is made into an extremely painful and therefore abnormal condition.

The cause of uterine pain in uncomplicated labour is, therefore, due to the condition of the interpretation of the sensations to which a woman is subjected. The false interpretation of these sensations sets up nervous impulses which give rise to excessive tension – which stimulates the nociceptors (receptors) placed there by nature to warn the patient of that condition. Then real pain supervenes. . . . The great intensifier of stimulus interpretation is fear. . . . Thus we have the three great evils: pain, fear and tension. It is this syndrome which is responsible for the pain of labour.

Dr Dick-Read – who, ·incidentally defines pain as 'a mental interpretation of injurious stimuli' – adds: 'If fear can be eliminated, pain will cease.'

Some midwives used to claim that pain was an essential part of labour: it gave the mother a feeling afterwards that she had really achieved something. But this philosophy has faded from medical practice in recent years and a great deal of effort is now put into preparing the minds of expectant mothers, in order to reduce ignorance and fear and so ease the pain of childbirth itself.

Some gynaecologists, notably in the Soviet Union, practise 'psychoprophylaxis', a kind of brain-washing technique in which the expectant mother is taught the physiology of the uterus and the mechanism of labour. She is encouraged to be aware of every little sensation during the birth, and to concentrate upon every detail of what is happening, so that her mind is fully occupied. Advocates of 'psychoprophylaxis' claim a 70 per cent success-rate in achieving 'painless' birth.

So, to sum up, pain is in the body – not always appearing early enough to be a 100 per cent reliable alarm (in cancer, for instance, it sometimes arrives too late) – but also in the mind. You can think yourself into pain, or out of it.

The mechanism of its behaviour seems to me to have similarities with computing. In computing, you have an 'input' – data which passes through teleprinters and is converted into signals which then travel along wires leading into the machine. With pain, you have an input, too – noxious stimuli which activate receptors to send signals along nerves leading to the spinal column and the brain.

In computing, you have a 'memory store', to which the fresh data can be related as it comes in. With pain you have a memory store, too: experience.

In computing, you have a 'processor' (for handling the data) and a 'programme', (for telling the machine how to handle it). The 'programme' controls the 'output' – in other words, the machine's reaction to the data. With pain, you have a processor also – probably two (one located in the spinal column, the other in the brain) – whose reactions to pain-data can be controlled, to a high degree, by the individual's own programme of wishes. If he wishes to ignore the pain, he may do so. If he wishes to suppress his reactions, he may sometimes be able to do that also.

Few people have learned to programme themselves to conquer pain. Most of us need a little help. And that is what the rest of this book is all about.

3

Some VIPs (Very Important Pains)

The courtyard was full of French soldiers, muddy and unshaven. One group was hurling corpses off the top of a pigsty; another was breaking down a stable door with the butts of their muskets. Upstairs, in the farmhouse itself, two shots rang out. A pair of German artillerymen had been discovered, cowering under a bed, and were summarily executed. From beyond the orchard, in the direction of an inn called La Belle Alliance, a continuous rumble of guns could be heard. The whole area was heavy with smoke. It was 6.30 p.m. and the evening was damp.

Near the right flank of the British line, the Duke of Wellington sat impassively on his horse. He was actually, at that moment, under fire. Musket-balls landed sporadically around him, kicking up little flecks of mud. From across the road leading to Nivelles a staff officer named Kennedy came riding up, just in time to hear the Duke say coolly: 'Drive those fellows away.' A posse of cavalry was dispatched to do so. The firing stopped.

Kennedy's news was bad. The farmhouse (known as La Haye Sainte and in the very centre of Wellington's line) had been overrun. Only 41 of the 360 Germans defending it had escaped. And the French seemed poised to attack again. . . .

Wellington felt that defeat was imminent. Thousands of his redcoats had been cut down by the French squadrons which had thundered into them, sabres flashing, lances thrusting. He had few reserves left.

Behind him, even the Household and Union Brigades of cavalry had had to be formed into a single, sprawling line to make them look thicker on the ground than they really were. Wellington knew that it needed only one more massive French assault to turn 18 June 1815 into one of the blackest days in British history, and he was quite sure that Napoleon was preparing to launch it.

But where was Napoleon?

The Emperor at that moment was perched on a mound near La Belle Alliance. Fortunately for the British, he could see very little. The whole of the ridge occupied by the thinned squares of Wellington's redcoats and the depleted cavalry, together with the crossroads where the Duke himself waited for German reinforcements, was obscured by smoke.

Had Napoleon reached the mound earlier in the day – before the gun-smoke had mingled with the mist to blot out the battlefield – he would certainly have appreciated the British plight and would probably have delivered the *coup de grâce*. But he was too late. He was late for the very good reason that he had spent a considerable part of the afternoon in pain, applying leeches to his anus – or rather to the haemorrhoids (piles) which were afflicting the rectal passage to his anus.

Napoleon was forty-five years old. Once lithe and vigorous – and always, as a commander, in the right place at the right time – he had grown fat, was frequently racked with pain, and exhibited from time to time a curious drowsiness which appeared to blunt his acuity and diminish his grasp of the strategic situation. He took care to hide his pain from his troops. Neither his doctor nor his personal valet revealed so much as a hint of his disability, and it was left to his brother, Prince Jerome, to release the secret several years after his death.

It is now known that not only did Napoleon suffer several acute attacks of piles during the battle of Waterloo but that he was a frequent victim of cystitis – inflammation of the bladder.

In his book *Waterloo – A Near-Run Thing* (Collins), the historian David Howarth comments:

> It was that inflammation of the bladder and urinary tract that had put him out of action at the battle of Borodino; he suffered from it many times before and afterwards, and it was found as a chronic condition in the post-mortem dissection at St Helena. It seemed to be brought on in acute attacks by cold and wet – and during the pursuit to Waterloo, the Emperor was soaked to the skin like everybody else.
>
> Cystitis can cause a high fever, and can also be very painful, with a constant need to pass water and acute pain when one does so – a pain which can absorb an ordinary person's attention and make him unable to concentrate his mind on anything else. If Houssaye's supposition was true [Henri Houssaye was an eye-witness], the piles had started on the night after [the battle of] Ligny, and the cystitis on the day after [the skirmish

at] Quatre Bras, and the Emperor, on the day of Waterloo, was suffering both these crippling kinds of pain and possibly had a fever – yet still had to try to direct his army, to force himself to think and be active, and to hide the pain and indignity from the thousands of men who were watching him.

Perhaps his brain was chronically less sharp than it had been: that must always remain a mere hypothesis. But whether it was or not, the passing effects of piles, cystitis and weariness are enough to account for everything he did or failed to do. He behaved that day like a sick man preoccupied with pain.

Pain is no respecter of persons. Napoleon apart, some Very Important People have had some very important pains.

On the morning of 24 June 1902, Albert Edward – second child and eldest son of Queen Victoria – was looking forward to his Coronation. Kings, queens, princes and princesses from far and wide had assembled in London. Stands had been erected along the processional route to Westminster Abbey. A feast of partridges, chickens, sturgeons and other delicacies – including 2,500 quail – had been ordered for the Coronation banquet.

Unfortunately, with only two days left to go, Edward and his queen gave a dinner party at Buckingham Palace for some of their guests. The menu was extravagant: consommé, whitebait, trout, quail, roast pullet, saddle of lamb, cold asparagus, salad, a punch gâteau laced with champagne, anchovy canapés and ice-cream, washed down by an 1892 Moët, a '74 Château Lango, George IV sherry and 1800 brandy. Afterwards, the royal couple chatted individually to all their guests before retiring.

That night, the king developed a sharp abdominal pain and a temperature. He had had recurring pain and discomfort for nearly a fortnight and his personal physician, Sir Francis Laking, in consultation with his Serjeant-Surgeon, Sir Frederick Treves, had diagnosed perityphlitis: appendicitis. But the pain and tenderness had subsided. The dinner party had been enough to bring it all back. At 10 a.m. on 24 June, Laking and Treves summoned three other specialists – Lord Lister, Sir Thomas Smith and Sir Thomas Barlow – and held a consultation at the king's bedside. Edward was all for carrying on with the ceremony.

'I must keep faith with my people,' he insisted, 'and go to the Abbey.'

'Then, sir, you will go in your coffin,' replied Treves.

Some three hours later Treves opened the king's lower abdomen. An operation for appendicitis, in those days, was still considered a

serious risk. The word appendicitis had not been invented until 1888
– indeed, Treves himself preferred the term 'recurrent typhlitis' –
and surgery was cautious.

The surgeon found a large abscess, from which he drained the pus
with the aid of two tubes. At 2 p.m., the following bulletin was
posted on the gates of Buckingham Palace: 'An operation on His
Majesty has been successfully performed. A large abscess has been
evacuated. The King has borne the operation well and is in a satisfactory condition.'

Sir Frederick Treves did not go to bed for seven nights, although
the royal appendix never actually had to be removed. The pain
subsided; the king recovered. A shortened Coronation ceremony
was held seven weeks later. The poor people of London enjoyed an
unexpected feast (the original ingredients for the Coronation banquet were distributed free) and the operation to relieve appendicitis
immediately became fashionable.

Other members of royal families have had to endure pain in common with their subjects.

In 1536, King Henry VIII of England was forty-five years old, a
domineering, whimsical and irascible man. He also had a leg ulcer.

Exactly what caused this leg ulcer is not known, but it was
certainly painful. Each time it healed up, Henry bellowed in pain.
The targets for his cries, in turn, were his third, fourth, fifth and
sixth wives, for pain seems to have struck most frequently in the
bedroom.

Several medical historians have speculated that Henry had syphilis
and that the ulcer was a *syphilitic gumma*, or inflamed tumour. James
Kemble, writing in the *Annals of Medical History*, considers that the
gumma may have penetrated to the marrow cavity and caused a
secondary infection – streptococcal osteomyelitis – which secreted
fluid constantly. Pain came whenever the only outlet for this secretion healed over. But Professor John Shrewsbury, in the *Journal of the
History of Medicine* suggests that it was due to uric arthritis of the
knee-joint, brought on by gluttony and heavy drinking.

On 26 January 1956, the Danish Medico-Historical Society met to
consider the medical problems of Henry VIII, who had died 409 years
previously. At the end of the meeting, Dr Ove Brinch summed up as
follows:

From the facts stated by other medical writers, as well as those
put forward by myself and the opinion of the specialists

expressed in the present discussion, it is possible to make the following diagnoses of the diseases of Henry VIII: (1) malaria; (2) obesity; (3) inebriety; (4) alcoholic polyneuritis; (5) tertiary syphilis (with multiple gummata); (6) secondary osteomyelitis; (7) alcoholic dementia and/or general paralysis of the insane; (8) psychopathy. Obviously it is impossible to diagnose syphilis with any certainty. . . . A scientific study of his bones would reveal the truth without any possible doubt.

But nobody seems willing to exhume poor Henry's bones; and perhaps he had reason to be grateful that only one of his many conditions caused him actual pain.

Queen Anne, last of the Stuarts to become sovereign of England, could not exactly be called a great beauty. She had smallpox at twelve, persistent inflammation of the eyes, and a short-sightedness which made her frown constantly. But her husband, Prince George, made her pregnant seventeen times before she was thirty-five.

Small wonder, then, that by the time Anne succeeded to the throne in 1702 she was virtually crippled, and in great pain. Only one of her children survived more than a few weeks of life – William – and he died at the age of eleven from hydrocephalus. She herself developed dropsy and gout, and at her coronation had to be carried in a low armchair and supported by the Lord Great Chamberlain and the Archbishop of Canterbury to reach the altar.

Anne was a glutton. She ate prodigiously – often a whole chicken to herself, with four or five courses before and several after. Eventually she developed gout in the stomach as well as in the legs.

Dean Swift, chronicler of his time, gave this description of her in 1713: 'The gout vibrated fearfully through the Queen's frame, flying from her feet to her stomach. At last, being carried in an open chair, on 9 April, to the House of Lords, Her Majesty pronounced her speech with her usual harmony of utterance, yet it was noted that her voice was weaker than usual.' By July, she was so corpulent that 'she had not been able to walk a step since the preceding November, and was obliged to be lifted into her coach by a machine that had been constructed for that purpose'. She also had a block and tackle fitted in Windsor Castle to lift her from room to room.

She died on 1 August 1714 and was buried in a coffin which was almost square. Yet she had never inflicted her pain on her people, and during her reign some of the best English architecture, drama, poetry and prose was created, not to speak of the English political party system.

In June 1788, King George III – longest-ever tenant of the English monarchy – summoned his doctors for a bedside consultation. He had spent a restless night, with severe abdominal pain. He had also passed urine which was coloured red. The physicians, without the benefit of stethoscope, thermometer or reflex hammer in those days, had only the king's verbal description to go by, coupled with whatever their fingers and eyes could detect in the region of the royal midriff. They diagnosed 'biliary Concretions in the Gall Duct'.

During the next two months, the king became highly excitable. His stomach pains returned in October, together with a stiffness of the limbs (diagnosed as 'rheumatism' and – when it particularly affected the legs – as 'gout'). Constipation and colic followed. By December, the king was in considerable pain, sweating, constantly, complaining of cramps, lameness and 'stitches in the breast', and unable to sleep. He began to have fits. Some considered him to have gone mad.

It was not the first time he had been so afflicted, nor was it to be the last. During his sixty years as monarch, medical historians have identified five separate, major attacks with similar symptoms, and four minor ones. Controversy has continued ever since his death in 1820 as to what was wrong with him. Possibly his early irritability and fits of temper were provoked by pain: in later years, he was clearly mentally deranged.

One explanation put forward to account for all the symptoms is porphyria – a rare, hereditary disease of the metabolism, characterized by the reddish colour of the urine. But the diagnosis is far from proven. Suffice to say that during the time the king was ill, his conduct of political affairs deteriorated and some nineteenth-century historians attributed directly to him the loss of the American colonies.

Severe pain seems also to have been a particular scourge of Presidents of the United States.

On 18 June 1893, Dr R. M. O'Reilly found a rough patch about the size of a coat button on the palate of the then President of the United States, Grover Cleveland, during a physical examination. He removed some tissue and sent it away for analysis without informing the pathologist of its origin.

Cancer was confirmed. Further examination showed that the malignant growth stretched from the left bicuspid teeth to within one-third of an inch of the soft palate, and had invaded the bone of the upper jaw.

America, at that time, was facing a crisis. The US Treasury was short of gold. It had been Grover Cleveland's intention to introduce a Bill to repeal what was known as the Sherman Silver Purchase Act, which made it compulsory for the Government to purchase silver, even at the expense of its gold reserve.

Had Cleveland not been able to, it is likely that America would have been forced on to a silver standard, rather than a gold standard. As the journal *The Commercial and Financial Chronicle* put it: 'Mr Cleveland is about all that stands between this country and absolute disaster: his death would be a great calamity.'

Little did the editor know how close to death the President had come. . . .

In fact, only eight men were let into the secret. The President knew that if Congress got to know that he had cancer of the jaw, confidence in his ability to carry through the proposed legislation would be sapped. He instructed his personal physician, Dr O'Reilly, to restrict the number of people who should be told of his condition to the handful needed to carry out immediate surgery. The President had a close friend, Commodore E. C. Benedict, who owned a yacht. It was decided to perform the operation aboard the yacht to minimize the risk of outsiders getting to hear of it.

On 30 June, three doctors, a surgeon and a dentist joined the President and Mr Benedict aboard the yacht *Oneida*, standing at Pier A in the Port of New York. The only other person present was Cleveland's political confidant, Secretary of War, Lamont. The yacht slipped moorings and headed for Bellevue Bay, where the President was given a thorough medical examination.

Next day, as the yacht moved slowly up New York's East River, the operation was performed. Dr O'Reilly administered nitrous oxide and ether, Dr Hasbrouck (the dentist) took out the two bicuspid teeth and Dr Joseph Bryant (one of the surgeons) cut clear the cancerous bone and some of the surrounding tissue. He was careful only to cut *inside* the mouth, so that no external scars would be left. Throughout the operation, the President remained propped up on pillows in the yacht's cabin. Despite the fact that he was fifty-six and corpulent he stood up to surgery remarkably well. Two days later he was up and about.

On 5 July, *Oneida* arrived off Cape Cod and dropped anchor in Buzzards Bay. The President had a summer residence there, Gray Gables, and he spent most of the next week sitting in the sun. Unfortunately, some of the gum-tissue close to the site of the cancer began to show signs of abnormality, and his physicians advised a second, minor operation.

He went back aboard the yacht. The operation was carried out at sea on 17 July and seems to have been a complete success. A New York dentist, Dr Kasson Gibson, fashioned a rubber prosthesis to pack out the President's face and make it look normal, and he resumed active public life early in August. The Sherman Silver Purchase Act was successfully repealed and America recovered its economic equilibrium.

When on 29 August the *Philadelphia Press* published an account of the operation, the President issued a signed statement denying it. It seems that Dr Hasbrouck, the dentist, accidentally 'leaked' the story to a medical colleague who in turn related it to a friend on the *Philadelphia Press*.

It was not until 22 September 1917 – nine years after Grover Cleveland had died (not from cancer but heart failure) – that a detailed account of the secret surgery was revealed in the *Saturday Evening Post*. The author was Dr W. W. Keen, a Philadelphia surgeon, and one of the eight men who had been present aboard the yacht.

Franklin D. Roosevelt was another American President who suffered more than his fair share of pain.

In 1914, as a Senator, he developed an acute appendicitis. In 1916 he had several attacks of tonsillitis, and in 1919 had his tonsils removed – 'not', as he put it, 'an agreeable operation'. But his life of pain did not really start until the night of 10 August 1921.

The Roosevelts – Franklin, Eleanor and their six children – had been sailing at Campobello, an island in New Brunswick, where they had a summer residence. On their way home, they saw flames sweeping through the trees on a neighbouring island. They dropped anchor and went ashore to fight the flames. Afterwards, Roosevelt swam in a lake to cool off and remove the soot, then went for a run. Later that evening, he swam again. Soon afterwards, sitting in his wet bathing costume reading his mail, he felt a sudden chill. 'I think I'll go to bed, dear,' he said to his wife.

Next morning he had a temperature of 103°F. and a sharp pain in his left leg. Mrs Roosevelt called in the local doctor.

The temperature subsided a little, but Dr E. H. Bennett remained concerned because Roosevelt could only walk with pain. The pain had also spread to his back.

By chance, there happened to be summering in the area an emin- ent surgeon – Dr W. W. Keen – who had actually been one of those in attendance during the jaw operation on President Cleveland twenty-eight years previously. Dr Bennett decided to call him in for consultation. Keen was then eighty-three. He diagnosed 'a clot of blood from a sudden congestion' which had 'settled in the lower spinal cord, temporarily removing the power to move but not to feel'. But a few days later, as Roosevelt's condition worsened, he changed his mind. 'A lesion of the spinal cord' was the next diagnosis, and he prescribed vigorous massage, delivering a bill for 600 dollars at the same time.

Vigorous massage was about the worst thing Roosevelt could have been given, for the Senator was actually suffering from poliomyelitis – or 'infantile paralysis' as it was then called – something which the aged Dr Keen had never seen.

Roosevelt's condition worsened further. He was in intense pain. He had to urinate through a tube because the sphincters – circular muscles – controlling the bladder and bowel were paralysed. After a fortnight, a specialist from Boston confirmed acute anterior poliomyelitis and ordered the massage to cease at once.

By mid-September, the specialist declared Roosevelt to be strong enough to be moved to hospital in New York, and a private railway-coach was hired to transport his stretcher with as little fuss as possible. But he was discharged from hospital on 28 October as 'not improving'.

A family squabble developed over his future: his mother, Sara Roosevelt, wanted him to give up politics and retire to a quiet life; his wife, Eleanor, thought that resumption of an active, political career might help him. Eleanor won. She wrote of his convalescence: 'Franklin's illness proved a blessing in disguise; for it gave him strength and courage which he had not had before. He had to think out the fundamentals of living and learn the greatest of all lessons – infinite patience and never-ending persistence.'

Later, one of his Cabinet colleagues, Frances Perkins, commented: 'Franklin Roosevelt underwent a spiritual transformation during the years of his illness. The years of pain and suffering had purged the slightly arrogant attitude Roosevelt had displayed before he was stricken. The man emerged completely warm-hearted with humility of spirit and a deeper philosophy.'

The Atlantic Ocean off south-west Spain that afternoon was rolling with a heavy swell. Although watchers ashore could see little, the rumble of cannon was unmistakable. Ten miles out to sea, two great fleets tossed and reeled, locked in mortal combat. Sixty-four ships in all, sails at the full, smashing life out of each other with iron, lead and fire. And everywhere, thick smoke.

The battle off Cape Trafalgar had begun just ten minutes before noon with a burst of shot from the French square-rigger *Fougeux*. But the rolling of the swell had sent the first cannon-balls high, barely touching the topsails of its target, *Royal Sovereign*.

It was the signal for all hell to be let loose. The French and Spanish fleets, strung out in line-ahead formation across four miles of ocean, soon found themselves split – !rst into three, then into smaller units – by compact driving lines of British ships employing impudent naval tactics.

Guns flared, grape-shot whistled through rigging, boarding-parties readied themselves with cutlasses and bayonets drawn. One by one, the groups of hostile fighting-ships grappled in the smoke until, finally, one or other lay wrecked, crews savaged, ensigns torn down, despair at capitulation mingling with the agony of the wounded.

At about 1.25 that fateful afternoon – 21 October 1805 – two ships in particular were moving towards each other, ready for their own personal fight to the death. One, the *Redoubtable*, had a fiery little commander less than five feet tall aboard, a Frenchman named Captain Lucas. The other, the *Victory*, carried the British commander-in-chief, Admiral Lord Nelson.

Lucas had made a special point, whenever his ship was in harbour, of training his men in the art of throwing grappling-irons and hand-grenades, and in musketry from the rigging: the French favoured hand-to-hand fighting, the British despised it.

Accordingly, as the *Victory* bore down on the *Redoubtable*, the tactics of the two commanders were at variance. Lucas wanted to board the British flagship from the tops. He had positioned more than a hundred musketeers and grenadiers in the rigging. Nelson was bent on blasting the hull, decks and masts of the *Redoubtable* to pieces with his fifty starboard guns, keeping the fight at water-level.

The *Victory* rammed into the port bow of the French ship, locked and swung. The flanks of the two warships came together. As they did so, the *Redoubtable* slammed her gunports shut and a hail of bullets and grenades poured down from her rigging. British tars, blue-and-white-striped vests bespattered with blood, fell by the dozen. Within minutes, fifty had been wounded or killed. Others manfully carried on loading the guns, loosing off fusillades as fast as their ramrods could press fresh shot up the barrels.

It was the practice of ships' officers at the time – and especially commanders – to show their contempt for their opponents by strutting up and down the decks, in full view of the enemy, with no regard for personal safety. Such displays of bravado inspired the sailors under their command to stay at *their* posts, under fire. Horatio Nelson was no exception. Although Lucas's musketeers could have been no more than forty feet from him, although his decks were splintered and pockmarked by grenades, although many of his men had been carried to the cockpit below, he continued to pace the quarter-deck – poop to hatch and back again – as if his ship were in the calm safety of Spithead on an English summer's afternoon.

It says little for the marksmanship of the French that it was twenty minutes before a musket-ball from up top struck the forepart of Nelson's epaulette, entered his left shoulder, descended obliquely through a lung, smashed through his spine and finally embedded itself in the lower muscles of his back. 'They have done for me at last,' he told Captain Hardy. 'Yes, my backbone is shot through.'

The *Victory*'s surgeon, Sir William Beatty – hard-pressed that day – recorded the final moments of the dying warrior some two months later. At the time, the flagship was sailing up the English Channel with Nelson's body, embalmed in a keg of rum to preserve it, ready for a State funeral. This was the surgeon's account:

> About the middle of the action with the combined fleets, on the 21 October last, the late illustrious commander-in-chief, Lord Nelson, was mortally wounded in the left breast by a musket-ball, supposed to be fired from the mizzen-top of the *Redoubt-able*, French ship-of-the-line, which the *Victory* fell on board of early in the battle; his Lordship was in the act of turning on the quarter-deck, with his face towards the enemy, when he received his wound; he instantly fell, and was carried to the cockpit, where he lived about two hours.
>
> On his being brought below, he complained of acute pain about the sixth or seventh dorsal vertebra, of privation of sense and motion of the body and inferior extremities; his respiration short and difficult; pulse weak, small, and irregular; he frequently declared his back was shot through; that he felt every instant a gush of blood within his breast; and that he had sensations which indicated to him the approach of death. In the course of an hour his pulse became indistinct, and was gradually lost in the arm; his extremities and forehead became soon afterwards cold. He retained his wonted energy of mind and exercise of his faculties until the latest moment of his existence; and when victory, as signal as decisive, was announced to him, he expressed his pious acknowledgements thereof and heartfelt

satisfaction at the glorious event in the most emphatic language; he then delivered his last orders with his usual precision,
and in a few minutes afterwards expired without a struggle.

Nelson was often in pain. Some of it may have been imaginary. An
examination of his medical history discloses a remarkable preoccu-
pation with his state of health throughout his life. But it is a fact that
he underwent more operations than any other flag-officer, and
Surgeon Commander P. D. Gordon Pugh, in his book *Nelson and
his Surgeons* has compiled a list of twenty-five doctors who attended
him at various times, although Nelson himself – in a letter to the
Duke of Clarence in 1794 – asserted: 'One plan I pursue, never to
employ a doctor: Nature does all for me and Providence protects
me.'

As a lieutenant, Nelson went down with malarial fever and
poisoning from eating manchineel leaves in the West Indies. As a
captain, he had scurvy and complained of pains in the chest and
lungs – possibly symptoms of tuberculosis, although they never
matured. In 1786, fever gripped him again and he became so fearful
of his life that he ordered a puncheon of rum (about seventy-two
gallons) to be prepared to receive his body (it was the practice, when
important people died at sea, to pickle their bodies in rum to preserve
them until they could be brought ashore for burial). Happily,
Nelson survived this episode.

1796 saw him complaining 'as if a girth were buckled taut over my
breast' and he gave an account of his 'endeavour in the night to get it
loose'. 1800 brought an attack of stomach pains of which he wrote:
'It is too soon to form an opinion whether I can ever be cured of my
complaint.' But he was.

A letter to the then Inspector-General of Hospitals in 1804
reported:

> I have had a sort of rheumatic fever, they tell me, but I have
> felt the blood gushing up the left side of my head, and the
> moment it covers the brain, I am fast asleep. I am now better of
> that; and with violent pain in my side, and night-sweats, with
> heat in the evening, and feeling quite flushed . . . the pain in
> my head, nor spasms, I have not had for some time.

On other occasions, Nelson complained of 'one of my terrible
spasms of heart-stroke which near carried me off' and of a sensation
as if his heart was actually 'breaking in two'. But at his post-mortem,
Sir William Beatty, the surgeon aboard the *Victory* who examined

his body, reported that his internal organs were so healthy that they 'rather resembled those of a youth than a man in his forty-eighth year'.

During the seige of Bastia in April 1794 Nelson received what he called 'a sharp cut in the back'. On 12 July, during the seige of Calvi, he recorded that he 'was much bruised about the face and eyes by sand from the works struck by a shot . . . a little hurt but not much'. But a month later, he was telling Lady Nelson that 'the blow was so severe as to occasion a great flow of blood from my head . . . my right eye nearly deprived of sight'. A court of examiners at the Royal College of Surgeons later declared that the injury was 'fully equal to the loss of an eye'.

At the battle of Cape St Vincent in February 1797, Nelson was officially listed as a casualty – 'bruised but not obliged to quit the deck' – and during the attack of Santa Cruz five months later, his right elbow was shattered by grapeshot. 'I am shot through the arm,' he cried, 'I am a dead man.' But thanks to the prompt action of his stepson, Josiah Nisbet, who was with him at the time and who improvised a tourniquet out of a handkerchief, his life was spared. The wounded Nelson was rowed back to HMS *Theseus* and, in the cockpit, had his arm amputated. Rum was the only anaesthetic, but he may have been given a leather pad to bite on. (As a result of this operation, Nelson ordered that a portable stove should be supplied to every ship in the fleet so that surgeons' instruments could be warmed.) Afterwards he was given opium to dull the pain.

Nelson was in pain for many months to come. Silk ligatures were used to sew up the stump of the arm and it seems that the surgeon somehow wrapped up the median nerve with one of the ligatures, so that each pull on it was agonizing. Eventually, on 3 December 1797, the offending ligature finally came away and Nelson sent a prayer of thanks to the rector of St George's, Hanover Square. It read: 'An officer desires to return thanks to Almighty God for his perfect recovery from a severe wound, and also for many mercies bestowed upon him.'

However, Nelson felt a 'phantom limb' pain in the stump of his right arm for the rest of his life. He suffered one more acute attack of pain before he was killed: on 1 August 1798, a piece of shot struck his forehead, causing a three-inch long wound and baring his skull. 'I am killed,' he cried again, 'Remember me to my wife.' But the message was unnecessary. Furthermore, while convalescing, he fell in love with Lady Hamilton and soon forgot his pain. . . .

★

There is no evidence that Nelson ever met 'John Taylor' during any of his visits to other ships in his fleet, nor indeed would he be likely to have paid particular attention to the youthful powder-monkey had he done so. Taylor looked like any other jolly Jack Tar. But beneath the striped vest and breeches of that particular servant of His Majesty lurked a secret: 'John Taylor' was a woman. She was, in fact, Mary Anne Talbot, the illegitimate child of the first Earl Talbot, born in 1778. Her story is included here because it is a remarkable example of a woman's ability to bear pain and to exert mind over matter. Mary was seduced, as a thirteen year old, by a particularly obnoxious captain in the 82nd Regiment of Foot, who thereafter forced her to dress as a boy and to accompany him on active service abroad – first to St Domingo, then to Flanders. Eventually, in 1792, her ravisher was killed by a musket-ball during the capture of Valenciennes.

Fearing further rape, Mary kept up her disguise and became a cabin-boy aboard a French lugger, which was subsequently captured in the Channel by the British Fleet. She was personally interviewed by the fleet commander, Lord Howe, and related all her story – merely omitting her sex. Howe believed it and arranged for the 'cabin-boy' to serve aboard the *Brunswick* as a powder-monkey, fetching and carrying powder and ammunition for the guns.

Unfortunately, on 1 June 1792 and during a spirited battle with French warships, Mary was wounded. A grape-shot struck an after-brace on a gun and ricocheted off the deck into her left leg, lodging just above the ankle and shattering the bone. She lay in excruciating pain for the remainder of the action, during which the ship's captain was killed, until transported by fellow sailors to the cockpit for medical treatment.

The ship's surgeon was unable to remove the shot for fear of injuring the tendons amongst which it was embedded. So for two days, until the *Brunswick* docked at Spithead, Mary lay biting back her moans of pain but trying to remain conscious for fear of revealing her secret in delirium.

She was taken to Haslar Hospital at Gosport, underwent surgery, continued to attend the hospital for four months as an outpatient and was finally discharged as 'partially cured', her secret still intact. But the pain recurred. She was forced to re-enter hospital – both the Middlesex and St Bartholomew's have her on record – but when surgeons finally decided to amputate her leg she discharged herself and limped out. She joined the frigate *Vesuvius* as part of Sir Sidney Smith's squadron, but was captured and imprisoned for eighteen months at Dunkirk. She finally escaped, only to be seized by a press-gang in Wapping. They tore the clothes off her and discovered her sex.

She was discharged by the Navy and eventually – after many applications – was granted a pension of twelve shillings a week in the name of John Taylor. But that was not the last of poor Mary. She formed a liaison with a notorious highwayman named Haines – who was subsequently hanged – and then went to work as a servant for a London publisher. She died at the age of thirty.

Sir Walter Scott was a prolific writer and many of his works – *The Waverley Novels*, *Guy Mannering*, *The Bride of Lammermoor*, *Ivanhoe*, *Redgauntlet*, to name but a few – are still widely read. But few people know that at the height of his literary career, Scott was afflicted by violent stomach cramps.

For four years – from 1817 to 1821 – he was frequently doubled up in pain, although the cause of it was never clear. He had recourse to opiates. It is said that he sometimes took as many as 200 drops of laudanum and six grains of opium a day. *The Bride of Lammermoor* is said to have been dictated by Scott when he was heavily under the influence of opiates because of his stomach cramps and it is probably for this reason that the author could not, subsequently, recognize much of the work as his own. He is said to have read the book after it was printed as though it had been written by someone else.

William Wilkie Collins's love of opium has already been mentioned earlier in this book. He began to take it in the early 1860s in order to relieve pain in his joints and eyes. Soon, he was taking copious quantities of laudanum. He is another who does not remember writing sequences in one of his books – *The Moonstone* – because he was under the influence of the drug.

Guy de Maupassant, on the other hand, believed that he wrote better if he had taken 'a little something' to relieve pain. In his case it was ether, inhaled to relieve severe and frequent headaches.

George Crabbe, who died in 1832, was another who suffered from headaches. He began working life as a surgeon-apothecary but, after four years of medical practice, left his home town – Aldeburgh in Suffolk – to become a poet in London. His works included *The Village*, *Tales of the Hall* and *The Newspaper* and Byron once described him as 'Nature's sternest painter – but the best'.

Crabbe turned to opium for relief from both the headaches and vertigo. He may well have been a victim of migraine.

The scene switches to an airfield in Wiltshire, England. It is 1943. The crew of a Lancaster bomber are in their places, carrying out cockpit checks. Down on the tarmac, a small group of senior officers and a civilian are huddled in conversation, coat-collars drawn up against the wind, hands rammed deep into pockets.

Abruptly, the civilian breaks away and walks quickly to a grey staff car. He does not get in but moves around the back and leans against the luggage compartment. He is feeling sick.

Inside the plane, pale-green lights pick out the helmeted faces of the crew, testing oxygen masks and intercoms. The ground crew check the latches on the bomb-bay doors and one of them steps back to give the 'thumbs up' sign. Great engines roar into life. The senior officers move back to the staff car where, by now, the civilian has composed himself. 'Flaps thirty! Radiators closed!' The Lancaster begins to move forward.

'Lock throttles – full power.' Some of the ground crew give a V-sign and from the rear turret there is a matching response. The Lancaster's nose tilts forward slightly, the tail assembly lifts clear of the ground and seconds later the great bomber is airborne, a strange cargo locked in its belly: a new bomb, called Tallboy.

'Excuse me,' the civilian says to his colleagues in the staff car, 'I must get out.' Pain grips the left side of his head in a vicious steel band. Spots have come before his eyes and vertigo makes him feel sick again. He gets out and goes behind the staff car once more.

His name is Barnes Wallis.

That scene – and many similar ones – became a familiar one to everybody who worked with Barnes Wallis on the development of the great dam-busting bombs, Tallboy and Upkeep, during the war. For Dr Wallis was a victim of migraine.

Migraine – probably recognized as long ago as 3,000 years BC and alluded to in an Egyptian papyrus as 'a sickness of half the head' – is characterized by a severe, one-sided headache, with blurred or partial loss of vision, and sometimes a feeling of pins and needles. Its symptoms and treatment are discussed more fully in the next chapter; suffice it to say here that in addition to Barnes Wallis it has afflicted such famous people as Joan of Arc, Pascal, Napoleon and Lewis Carroll.

Sir Barnes, when I saw him in 1975 after his eighty-seventh birthday, told me that although migraine did not actually halt his work he lost about twenty-four hours of working time a fortnight because of it. This, in total, meant a year of his life. He first experienced the pain at the age of twelve: 'The whole school used to lunch together,' he told me,

. . . and in the Great Hall there was a beautiful pulpit – on the side of the hall – in which one of the senior boys would stand to say grace after the meal. All the school would turn to face the pulpit. I can well remember looking at the boy, and his suddenly disappearing from view: that was my first experience. I thought I'd been struck blind or something dreadful had happened.

It really is quite an uncomfortable and an alarming thing, and a set of violent pins and needles in your tongue, or in your fingers, or right down to your big toe, are most unpleasant and very realistic to the sufferer, although the onlooker can see nothing the matter with you at all.

During the war, when I was working in the New Forest developing the Tallboy and the Upkeep bombs for dam-busting, and travelling back from Salisbury, I really think I was sick in every ditch – a most unpleasant sensation because people look at you being sick, hiding behind the back of your car as well as you can, and think you're probably a drunk or something of that sort!

'Unbutton your blouse!'

She undid the two top buttons. The man behind her drew her blouse back so that the corrugations of her spine were bare. On the third vertebra he laid a red-hot poker.

'Where is Arnaud?'

'I have nothing to say.'

'My colleague here, Lise, is going to pull out your toe-nails, one by one, starting at the little toe of your left foot.'

She felt him take her left foot in his hand and felt the steel jaws of the pincers settle tightly around the tip of her nail. With a slow, muscular drag he began to pull.

'Now would you care to tell me Arnaud's address?'

The above conversation and incident are still clear in the mind of Mrs Odette Hallowes, GC, another who has vivid memories of pain suffered during the 1939–45 war. Mrs Hallowes – the wartime agent Odette Sansom – was tortured by the Gestapo at their headquarters near Fresnes prison, Annecy, in May 1943. On that particular occasion, she lost all ten of her toe-nails. At other times she was beaten, burned, kicked and flogged. But she refused to divulge information which the Germans wanted, preferring instead the pain.

Almost thirty-two years later, she told me:

I was not especially brave. I simply tried to live from moment to moment, saying to myself 'You've got through that moment of pain, now you can get through the next', and feeling a sense of achievement at having endured each pain. You never know what you can do until you try, but the human body is capable of surprising things; it is quite amazing, the power it holds. I was helped quite a bit by my surroundings: the prison had trees outside, which I could see through the window. When they were doing things to me I thought about the trees and the fact that it was early summer and lovely weather. Peace comes to you when you least expect it.

Odette added: 'Of course, you mustn't be selfish; you must accept the supreme sacrifice. You must be prepared to die, then death has no sting. It hasn't for me any more. It will come to me one day as a friend.'

Iain Macleod, Conservative·MP for Enfield West for twenty years, was in considerable pain for most of them. He suffered from spondylitis – inflammation of the vertebrae – which, around 1959 when he was appointed Colonial Secretary, became ankylosed. His neck became more and more rigid and he was forced to resort more and more to pain-killers to keep going.

Three years after his death in July 1970, I asked his widow, Baroness Macleod of Borve, whether pain had ever impaired his judgement. 'His judgement', she answered,

. . . was only impaired, in my view, on two occasions – but both of them were due to our daughter being desperately ill and not by the pain itself. Once his neck had set rigid, and that caused him more embarrassment than actual pain because he could not raise his head to see anybody unless he bent his whole body backwards. It was, therefore, much easier for him to speak to an audience from a high platform – such as at party conferences – than from the floor of the House, where he had to swivel on his heels to see the Members.

Lady Macleod went on: 'I cannot remember a single occasion when he had to succumb to pain and miss an appointment, although he was frequently tired through lack of sleep due to pain the previous night. He took pills to help him sleep and also pain-killers, but he learned to live with pain. Some people can accept it while others are worn down.'

She added: 'Despite the ups and downs of fortune and health, I am sure my husband enjoyed his life. Pains did not prevent him from doing so.'

The morning of Monday, 14 December 1931 was bright, clear and crisp. On the grass of Woodley Aerodrome in Berkshire, three Bristol Bulldog fighter-planes were drawn up in front of the clubhouse, parked in a neat 'V', wings glinting.

In the warm, slightly steamy lounge, a group of young pilots were drinking coffee and asking questions of a stocky, square-jawed flier in overalls, perched on the arm of a chair. His name: Douglas Robert Stewart Bader. Rank: Pilot Officer, RAF.

Bader was only twenty-one. But already he had become something of a hero to fellow pilots because of his dare-devil manoeuvres as part of the RAF aerobatics team, then based at Kenley. On this particular morning, all the questions were about aerobatics.

Somebody suggested a 'beat-up' of the airfield. Bader declined. The conversation switched but as they were about to leave, another pilot revived the idea. Again Bader said 'No'.

He remembers hearing some mutterings and the word 'windy'. He remembers striding, tight-lipped, to the Bulldog. He remembers taking off, banking steeply and roaring in towards the clubhouse, just grazing the boundary fence; the roll to the right; the flip over; the feel of the stick in his hands as he rolled again to the right. He remembers a terrible noise; and then nothing.

The left wing-tip of the Bulldog had hit the grass, jerking the nose down. The propeller had gouged out a huge furrow, the cowling had exploded and torn the engine out by its roots. The rest of the plane had cartwheeled, shattered and crumpled. Somewhere in the tangle of wreckage, the young Bader – tipped as a likely fly-half for England in the coming international rugby season – had escaped. Or almost.

Paul Brickhill, whose biography of Bader, *Reach for the Sky* (Collins) was published in 1954, says the pilot recalls everything going suddenly quiet and still. 'The cockpit was tilted,' he goes on. 'That was odd. But it was only a hazy idea and not very interesting because pain was stabbing his back. Slowly it ebbed, leaving a passive torpor, and sitting in the straps, hands in his lap, he was placidly aware of the cockpit: beyond that, nothing.'

There was plenty more pain to follow. Leonard Joyce, one of the best surgeons in England at the time, removed first his right leg, then his left. Again, Brickhill recalls:

The [left] leg kept on hurting keenly and remorselessly. Sister Thornhill gave him a little morphia to ease it, but it seemed to make no difference: the terrible hurting went on, stabbing stronger and stronger till it was shredding his nerves all over and beginning to obsess him with agony. . . . Thornhill gave him more morphia but the pain went relentlessly on. . . . By nightfall his eyes were sunken and restless in dark hollows, and the face was grey and waxy, glistening with a film of sweat. For a while he slept under more morphia. . . . Later, the young man woke and the pain had gone.

But it was only temporary relief. Bader was in agony for a week, so overwhelmed by it that he could scarcely hold a conversation with visitors. There was a different pain – chafing and more stinging – after he was fitted with artificial legs. It continued, on and off, for months.

Yet when in 1975 I asked Group Captain Douglas Bader, DSO, DFC – the 'legless hero' of the Battle of Britain, as he was subsequently dubbed – to talk about his pain, he replied: 'I can't really help, I'm afraid. You see, it all happened forty-four years ago. I can remember that it hurt like hell but I can't actually relive it. You see, the great thing about pain is that you don't remember.it afterwards.'

He paused for a moment, then added: 'That's how women manage to go on having babies.'

4

The First Pain-Killers

The Land Rover looked like any other which had been on a long journey: dusty, caked with mud around the wheels, untidy in the cabin and reeking of a mixture of well-worn leather and human sweat.

'Good trip?' The customs officer's question brought a casual 'Not bad' from one of the occupants but silence from the others. 'Mind if I look inside?'

The three young men in bush jackets and denim slacks got out. 'Be our guest,' said the driver and, as the customs officer mounted, he noticed the words 'Trans-Asia Expedition' painted on the side of the door. He decided to call for assistance.

Three more customs men emerged from a hut at the dockside and systematically, over the next forty-five minutes, they checked every inch of the vehicle. They lifted the floor, examined the hood, measured and tapped the wheel arches, probed the petrol tank, dismantled the headlamps and tail-lights and even blew up the exhaust pipe.

Seats, map compartment, ventilation ducts, spare tyre – every crevice which might have contained smuggled contraband was carefully probed. Then, with the bonnet raised, they checked the engine. Everything looked normal, a heavy layer of oily grime covering everything, just as one might expect after a journey overland from Istanbul.

Or *almost* everything. Something caught one of the customs officers' eyes. The six filler plugs on the top of the battery seemed unusually white. He reached to unscrew one but it would not turn. Quickly the customs men dismantled the battery housing. As they did so, the electric leads clattered against the engine: they had never been connected. They were false. The real leads led away from the starter motor towards the chassis, where a second battery had been cunningly mounted.

The customs men lifted the first 'battery' on to the tarmac and examined it. They could see now that the whole box divided into two and they prised the two halves apart. Inside, packed neatly together and individually wrapped, were more than 200 brown-coloured sticks: opium.

Opium must rank with aspirin as being the most widely used drug of all time. It not only induces lethargy and sleep, it also relieves pain – although for more than 5,000 years nobody understood why.

The first reference to opium – contained in the juice of the poppy – seems to have been an inscription carved on a tablet by a member of the Sumerian tribe around 4000 BC. The Sumerians, who invented the oldest written language still in existence today, inhabited southern Mesopotamia and they used a special mark on some of their tablets – 'HUL GIL'. Hul is thought to have meant joy and Gil plants.

The ancient Egyptians certainly knew about plants that could bring joy. Fields of poppies grew so thickly around the town of Thebes that at one time opium acquired the alternative name 'thebecium'. Otherwise, the Egyptians called it 'spnn' and the poppy itself 'spn'. One extract from the famous Ebers Papyrus in Egypt – thought to have been scribed around 1550 BC – offers parents a delectable remedy for stopping their children crying: 'spnn of spn, together with flies' excrement, scraped from a wall, worked into a paste and put through a sieve. Drink for four days.'

The ancient Assyrians also seem to have used opium widely, both as a soporific and a pain-killer. They called the poppy juice 'pa pa' or sometimes 'lion fat' and they ate the roots of the plant as well, believing it to be an aphrodisiac. In a list of 115 vegetable potions, drawn up on tablets by some Assyrian priest in the seventh century BC, reference to opium is made no less than 42 times.

In Greek mythology, the poppy was dedicated to four deities: Nax (Goddess of Night), Thanatos (God of Death), Hypnos (God of Sleep) and Morpheus (God of Dreams). In one of the most famous of Greek legends, Demeter, deeply respected for her connections in high places in the world of agriculture, had lost her daughter Persephone. The fact that Persephone was the result of an incestuous relationship with her brother made no difference: she was a lovely girl and Demeter missed her. She inquired everywhere. Eventually, some eyewitnesses told her that the earth had literally opened and swallowed Persephone up. Demeter was heartbroken. She wandered forlornly about Greece until one day she came to the city of Sicyon, on the Peloponnesus and not a hundred miles from the Gulf of Corinth.

Growing in a meadow were some white and purple flowers. Some had large, flexible capsules on top. Out of curiosity, Demeter picked a few and slit them open. Out of the sunripe seed-cases oozed milky white liquid, which rapidly turned brown and congealed. She licked her fingers. Within minutes, a strange feeling of contentment spread over her. She forgot her sorrows. She forgot Persephone. She went into a deep sleep. . . .

The Greeks, who always had a name for everything, called the milky white fluid which Demeter had sampled 'opion'. It was, of course, the juice of the poppy – raw, untreated opium.

Quite apart from the legend of Demeter, Greek literature is riddled with references to opium. Statues and drawings of Demeter (who eventually persuaded her incestuous brother Zeus to rescue their bastard daughter from Hades and return her to her mother for two-thirds of each year) frequently portray her with a poppy in her hand. Even the unfortunate Persephone is said to have been gathering poppies when she was swallowed up. The seed-pod also appears on many pieces of Grecian pottery.

In real-life Greece in the fourth century BC, Hippocrates – more famous today for his oath – prescribed poppy wine as a medicine, calling it a 'hypnotic meconion' and recommending it for uterine infections.

Galen, who contributed so much to our understanding of pain, was perhaps the first physician to make really intelligent use of opium to treat a range of medical conditions. He lived from AD 130–200 but his favourite opiate – 'mithridate' – continued in use for more than fifteen centuries.

The Romans knew a lot about opium – both from Galen and from Dioscorides, an army surgeon in Nero's time, who wrote a comprehensive compendium of drugs which listed opium as both a sedative and a pain-killer. Unfortunately, the poppy-juice was also widely distributed by quacks, and thousands of Romans became addicted before its drawbacks were recognized.

It was the Arabs who were responsible for the spread of opium after the fall of Rome – first to Persia, then to the area which is now Malaysia, then to India. Opium was first mentioned in Persian literature in the sixth century AD but was probably in use earlier; unfortunately, the early Persians left no records save their sacred books. The Arab word for opium is 'af-yun'. The Arab doctor Avicenna – another important contributor to our understanding of pain – became so obsessed by it that he died in 1037 from opium intoxication.

The use of opium in the Middle Ages was fostered by travellers who gave romantic accounts of drug-taking after visiting Asia Minor. One of these travellers was Marco Polo. Although he does not refer specifically to opium in his *Travels*, he is strongly suspected of having been influential in its spread. Venice, the city to which Marco Polo repeatedly returned, was the hub of trade for all Europe at the time. Explorers scoured Asia not only for opium and similar narcotics but for aphrodisiacs and other medicines as well. Traders would move overland by camel, across Asia and up the Persian Gulf or Red Sea, and then unload their goods off the camels' backs at Levantine ports. Italian vessels would then ship them to Venice or Genoa for distribution throughout Europe.

Some opium undoubtedly came to Britain in this way, although it may well have been introduced originally by the Romans. Certainly, the crusades of the eleventh, twelfth and thirteenth centuries appear to have stepped up interest in opium, perhaps because many of the crusaders themselves adopted Arab customs.

One eleventh-century English remedy speaks of a 'soporific sponge' steeped in a mixture of opium, mandragora, hemlock, ivy, hyoscyamus, mulberry juice and lettuce, which could be inhaled. The sleeper was revived by applying fennel-juice to his nostrils.

In the thirteenth century, a pseudo-physician named Michael Scott suggested this prescription for surgeons: 'Take of opium, mandragora and henbane, equal parts. Pound and mix them with water. When you want to saw or cut a man, dip a rag in this and put it to his nostrils: he will soon sleep so deep that you may do as you wish.'

The problem was that sometimes he slept *too* well. . . .

PREPARING OPIUM

Opium, first of the great pain-killers, acts by depressing the central nervous system. It slows down mental activity. It produces a dream state which can be both pleasant and unpleasant.

Thomas De Quincey, who wrote *Confessions of an Opium Eater* in 1822, said that at first it made him feel in harmony with life. But later he began to get 'noonday visions' and had dreams of wild beasts and phantoms so that he 'awoke in struggles and cried aloud "I will sleep no more".'

As a drug of pleasure, it was originally eaten – or drunk, like tea, as an infusion. But for the past 200 years it has also been smoked, sniffed and injected. About 1,200 tons are produced each year licitly, and probably twice as much illicitly.

It comes from the species of poppy known as *papaver somniferum,* an annual which grows between two and four feet high and produces flowers with four petals. These may be white, pink, red, violet or purple, but are usually white. The leaves are large, smooth and green with a silvery sheen. The flowers last only a few days but they produce a central pod or capsule about the size of a hen's egg. About ten days after the petals have fallen, the capsule is lanced so that a milky, viscous fluid oozes out. As it dries, the fluid turns brown and hardens. It can then be scraped away into bowls. The capsule can be slashed repeatedly, but the narcotic content of the fluid becomes weaker with each slashing.

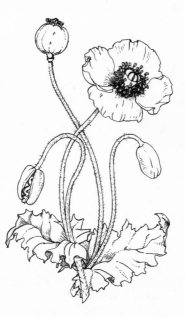

Opium poppy (*Papaver somniferum*)

As it dries harder, so the opium becomes darker. It is rolled into balls, each weighing about a pound, which have a rather sickly smell – rather like ammonia or stale urine – and a very bitter taste. It is made into cakes or bricks.

Raw opium can be produced almost anywhere; indeed, this is one of the problems in controlling its use. *Papaver somniferum* will grow quite happily in an English garden, although it prefers a dry climate.

Today it is grown prolifically in Turkey, Afghanistan, India, Pakistan, Thailand, Burma, Laos, Vietnam and Japan. Some is also grown in Russia, Bulgaria and Yugoslavia.

The raw opium is prepared for human use either by cooking it or by fermentation. It may be shaped into sticks – usually about seven inches long – slabs or blocks, and packed into tins or pots.

There are several forms of it. The form used for smoking is first boiled, evaporated and then toasted. A small lump is rolled between the fingers, or held between tongs or on a pin, and roasted over a flame. It is then pressed into the bowl of a pipe which, in turn, can be warmed over a flame or bed of glowing charcoal.

The smoker lies back and inhales deeply. The effect is immediate and each pipeful lasts about a minute. It produces a distinctive, sweet smell, but less tangy than marijuana.

The residue is known as 'burnt' opium and may either be mixed with fresh opium for the next pipe or mixed with water, boiled and then filtered. The solid material obtained is known as opium 'dross' and looks like little bits of charcoal. It is often sold to poorer smokers but it is highly toxic and usually leads to an early death.

There are opium dens today in China, Hong Kong, Shanghai, Malaya, Vietnam and even – it is said – in London, although I personally have been unable to find one.

In medicine, it is still used in the treatment of intestinal and renal colic, diarrhoea, rectal and pelvic pain, haemorrhoids, and even for colds and coughs. Martindale's *Extra Pharmacopoeia* lists twenty preparations which still contain it, including linctuses, tinctures, syrups and pastilles.

But it has had a chequered history.

THE CHINESE AND OPIUM

Many people associate opium with the Chinese. Indeed, there have been suggestions that the Chinese were the first to use it – ancient warriors were supposed to have been given it to suppress their fear of battle – but this now seems unlikely.

China does not appear to have been introduced to opium until the ninth century, and then only through trade with the East Indies. *Papaver somniferum* was grown primarily for ornamental purposes although there is evidence that opium was used in medicines as a remedy for dysentery. The Chinese called it 'ye pien' or 'o-fu-yung'. Curiously enough, it was the British who introduced them to the real horrors of opium.

Towards the end of the eighteenth century, Britain – through the medium of the British East India Company – was farming opium in a big way. Vast tracts of Bengal, Benares and Bahar were given over to poppy-growing, and the opium was sold to Malaya and the Dutch East Indies in return for tin and pepper.

It was also sold to China to allow Britons to indulge in a new passion, the drinking of China tea. In order to pay for the tea, the British bartered opium.

A British ship delivered the first consignment of the East India Company's opium to Canton in 1781. The Chinese called it 'Foreign Black Mud'. The Cantonese authorities attempted to legislate against it but the decrees were flouted by merchants of both sides; many officials were bribed to turn a blind eye.

Chinamen in Canton – and elsewhere in China – took to opium readily. It helped them to forget their poverty, bad food, poor housing, miserable existence and corrupt administration. Smoking dens sprang up everywhere. So did smuggling, robbery and a host of secret societies. Within ten years, opium was accounting for one quarter of all the trade between India and China.

In 1793, the Earl of McCartney was sent to China as an ambassador to try to set up proper trading rights between the two countries. Unfortunately, he was met with disdain by the Emperor, Ch'ien Lung. Ch'ien Lung would not even see him but sent back instead a letter addressed to George III – a yellow scroll wrapped in yellow silk lying on a yellow chair, tied to the back of a mandarin.

Part of it read: 'As your Ambassador can see for himself, we possess all things. I set no value on objects, strange or ingenious, and have no use for your country's manufactures.' Nevertheless, a limited amount of trade was eventually agreed to.

The official opium merchants had a tough time negotiating sales. There was no fixed tariff. Prices fluctuated daily. They were not allowed to learn Chinese and had no rights if they were arrested. However, trade in opium grew over the next thirty years, during which the Chinese turned to paying for it in silver as well as in tea. By 1833, according to American estimates, the British were getting twelve million dollars a year for their opium. Huge profits were made. Millions of people became addicted. Skulduggery was ubiquitous and dockside brawls between British and Chinese traders were an almost daily occurrence. Secret societies flourished. Canton and South China became virtually uncontrollable, and the Chinese government realized that it must act to stop its position being undermined further by the drain on its currency.

It did, in 1838. On the orders of Emperor Tao Kuang, a commissioner called Lin Tse Hsu was dispatched to Canton to stop the opium trade. Somehow he managed to persuade the Chinese traders to surrender their stocks and they handed over 20,000 chests of opium, 160lb of the drug in each chest. The British were furious. Under pressure from the East India Company, Lord Palmerston sent an expeditionary force to blockade Canton. Several cities fell to its assault and the Chinese – without a navy – found themselves in a hopeless position, with British East India Company ships able to fire with impunity on Chinese junks.

In 1842, the 'Opium War', as it has been called, came to an end. A treaty was signed in Nanking. Under it, the Chinese agreed to open five ports for trade of all kinds (Canton, Foochow, Shanghai, Amoy and Ningpo) and to give Hong Kong to the British. They also agreed to pay compensation for destroyed opium stocks. The opium trade resumed.

Getting the imperious Chinese to fulfil their obligations under the treaty, however, proved difficult and in 1856 further fighting broke out which lasted – on and off – for four years. During this time, Peking was captured and the opium trade legalized.

In 1907 China began negotiations with India to stop sending opium. Trade finally ceased on an official basis, although illicit opium trafficking continued. Unfortunately, when the Japanese invaded the Chinese mainland a few years later they used opium on a wide scale to try to get the submission and co-operation of the people.

Today, the mainland of China is once again free of opium addiction: at least, no Westerner can prove otherwise. A new opiate has taken its place: the thoughts of Chairman Mao.

UNDER THE INFLUENCE OF OPIUM

A great vogue for taking opium for pleasure grew up in Britain during the eighteenth and nineteenth centuries. It could be purchased openly, either in the form of a pill or as an ingredient of laudanum, a mixture of opium and alcohol.

Women drank it instead of brandy, men bought it because it was cheaper than gin, mothers even gave it to their babies. George IV was given it to stop stomach irritation, Clive of India died of it; even William Wilberforce took it for the last forty-five years of his life.

Writers of the time believed it stimulated artistic creativity. Coleridge was hooked on opium for a while. He started taking it in 1796 when he became aware of heart disease. By 1802 he was taking 100 drops of opium a day. Later he cut this to 12–20 drops and only took it when withdrawal symptoms became unbearable; his nightmares were often accompanied by screams which roused the whole household.

Coleridge was in contact with a literary network which regularly held opium sessions. There was no problem in obtaining the substance. In one of his Collected Letters, the poet records that one druggist in Thorpe was selling two to three pounds of opium a day and a gallon of laudanum. Much of *The Ancient Mariner* was probably written under the influence of opium and at the end of one version of *Kubla Khan* there is the note: 'This fragment, with a good deal more not recoverable, composed in a sort of reverie brought on by opium.'

Wilkie Collins, the novelist, was led to opium through a chance remark made by his mother to Coleridge. Coleridge had confided in her the difficulties he was having weaning himself off the drug. Mrs Collins replied: 'Mr Coleridge, do not cry. If the opium really does you any good and you must have it, why do you not go and get it?' Wilkie, then a young lad, overheard the remark and later witnessed his father dying, the only relief from pain being provided by opium. Small wonder that when he developed rheumatism in 1860 he himself turned to opium.

Collins never went anywhere later in life without his silver flask of laudanum. Opium began to creep into his novels – *No Name*, *Armadale* and finally *The Moonstone*. The latter – often described as the first detective novel – has a plot in which the precious moonstone is unwittingly stolen under the influence of opium and clues are uncovered by an opium-eater, portrayed as prematurely old, with sunken eyes, deep hollows in his cheeks and many wrinkles. He describes in the book his nights 'with the vengeance of the opium pursuing me through a series of dreadful nights'. But he claims to have needed opium to overcome ten years of terrible pain from disease, and it is interesting to see how Wilkie Collins persuades the characters who disapproved of this opium-taking to change their attitude in the end.

Wilkie Collins's friend, Charles Dickens, took opium occasionally, and actually went to an opium den. His experiences are woven into the character of Jasper, the murderer, in *The Mystery of Edwin Drood*, and the scene in the den is described like this:

He is in the meanest and closest of small rooms. Through the ragged window curtains, the light of early day steals in from a miserable court. He lies, dressed, across an unseemly bed, upon a bedstead that has indeed given way under the weight on it. Lying, also dressed and also across the bed, not longwise, are a Chinaman, a Lascar and a haggard woman. The two first are in a sleep or stupor; the last is blowing at a kind of pipe, to kindle it. And as she blows, and shading it with her lean hand, concentrates its red spark alight, it serves in the dim morning as a lamp to show him what he sees of her. 'Another?' says this woman in a querulous, rattling whisper. 'Have another?'

Earlier, Dickens had introduced opium – or rather laudanum – into the plot of *Oliver Twist*. Nancy uses it to drug the fearsome Bill Sykes so that she can escape to a meeting with Oliver's aunt, Rose Maylie, to tell her of Oliver's plight.

Byron turned to opium when his marriage broke up. He called it 'black drop'. Shelley took it for nervous headache, Lamb for a bad cold. Crabbe, poet and clergyman, started on it in middle age as a remedy for vertigo, and Keats – once apprenticed to a surgeon – refers to it in 'Ode to a Nightingale' in the following terms:

> My heart aches and a drowsy numbness pains
> My sense, as though of hemlock I had drunk,
> Or emptied some dull opiate to the drains,
> One minute past and Lethe-wards had sunk.

In 1830, Britain imported 22,000lb of opium. During the next thirty years, the quantity quadrupled. An 'opium sickness' pervaded society. Anyone addicted to it was not looked upon as indulging in a serious vice but merely in the same way as a person might be looked on today as having 'a drinking problem'.

Adults took it both as a narcotic and a pain-killer and children were given it through medicines with innocuous titles like 'Godfrey's Cordial', 'Dalby's Carminative', 'Munn's Elixir' or 'Mother Bailey's Quieting Syrup'. Many children are known to have died from overdoses, especially in the poorer quarters of cotton-spinning towns where mothers gave it to their babies when they had to go out to work.

In 1832, an American doctor named W. G. Smith recorded: 'There is scarcely a disease in which opium may not, during some of its states, be brought to bear by the judicious physician with advantage.'

It was not surprising. There were not many effective alternatives.

The Mysterious Mandrake

To the Egyptians, yet again, must go the credit for recognizing another of the early pain-killers: mandragora, or mandrake root. It seems to have been in use as long ago as the fourteenth century BC.

The two-pronged root was seen by some to resemble the human

form. Perhaps for this reason many legends and superstitions grew up around it. One of these was that it shrieked whenever it was touched (this may have had its origins in the fact that the mandrake sometimes grew beneath gallows and was said to feed on the flesh of criminals).

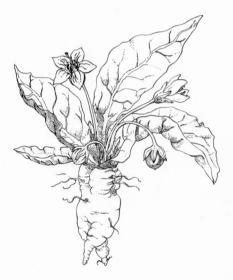

Mandrake (*Mandragora officinarum*)

Shakespeare alluded to it in *Romeo and Juliet*: 'And shrieks like mandrakes torn out of the earth, that living mortals, hearing them, run mad.' He also made a reference to it in *Antony and Cleopatra*: 'Give me to drink mandragora.'

The mandragora plant is one of the potato family and produces purple, bell-shaped flowers with a fleshy, orange-colour berry. In addition to being a narcotic, it also purges the bowels and can be used as an emetic to make people sick. It was used occasionally during the Middle Ages as a sedative before operations, but it frequently produced toxic side-effects and was administered with some trepidation.

The active ingredients in mandragora which can induce a kind of 'twilight sleep' have now been identified. They are atropine and scopolomine. Scopolomine – which has a numbing effect on parts of the central nervous system − is also present in another early analgesic, henbane. Apart from its pain-killing properties, it was thought to improve fertility and was used in many love-potions − and indeed, in the East it still is.

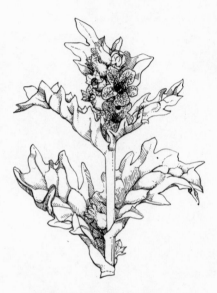

Henbane (*Hyoscyamus niger*)

Henbane

Henbane was said to have 'with invisible force pressed the eyelids shut'. Its botanical name is *Hyoscyamus niger* and it grows wild in Britain, chiefly on waste ground or rubbish dumps. Under the influence of concoctions obtained from its grey-green leaves, saints are said to have seen visions and soothsayers delivered oracles. Surgeons used it in the Middle Ages to deaden pain.

Unfortunately, the plant is also poisonous. It can trigger wild visions, even in the waking state, and frequently drove those who took it mad. Ancient alchemists were unable to separate the desirable ingredients from the dangerous and so, like mandragora, it was used with trepidation by medical men.

Today, however, henbane is used extensively in the preparation of atropine (a paralysing drug frequently given to dilate the pupils in eye examinations and to prevent muscle spasms), hyoscyamine (often prescribed for women who suffer painful periods) and hyoscine (also known as scopolomine, and swallowed by thousands of travellers each year to prevent sea-sickness).

Martindale's *Extra Pharmacopoeia* contains a list of thirty-six modern remedies involving henbane, which is grown commercially for medical purposes in Hungary, the Soviet Union, Egypt, France and the United States.

Henbane tea is still drunk in India and the seeds – which contain a higher proportion of hyoscyamine than the foliage – are sometimes sucked as a remedy (a highly dangerous one) for toothache. Unfortunately, as so often happens, hyoscyamine has also found its way into illicit smoking mixtures.

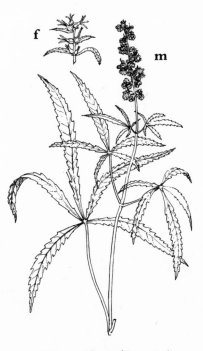

Hemp (*Cannabis sativa*)

Hashish

Cannabis – hashish, bhang, marijuana, pot, call it what you will – grows wild in many parts of the world. It is said to have been used in China 2,000 years ago to relieve pain during operations, but its use since has been mostly confined to those wishing to escape into a dreamworld of conscious drowsiness.

It has often been associated with crime and madness. In Marco Polo's day it was in widespread use in Asia Minor and, as a result of encountering one particular example of its evils, he is said to have introduced a new word into the language: 'assassin'. The story goes that Polo encountered some robbers operating out of mountains near Damascus. They were working for a sheikh who had originally lured them to his garden and plied them with hashish. Under the hallucinogenic influence of the drug, the garden suddenly appeared very beautiful – indeed, the young men described it as Paradise – but the sheikh would only allow them to remain there and take more hashish if they agreed to do his bidding. He trained them to rob, plunder and kill. The Arabic word for a drinker of hashish is 'hassassi', hence 'assassin'.

Perhaps the most reputable use of hashish was by the French army in the sixteenth century when it was given during battlefield operations.

Alcohol

Alcohol is another pain-reliever which has been in use since earliest times, probably since man first discovered that the fermented juice of berries or grain made him less aware of the world, able to sleep more deeply, and numb to the touch of others.

The Jews and Romans gave wine to the condemned before they went to the cross – Jesus got vinegar as a mockery – and even today, primitive tribes still intoxicate those selected for painful rituals.

Legend has it that Helen of Troy threw a substance into a crock of wine 'to quiet all pain and strife, and bring forgetfulness of every ill'. The substance is reputed to have been nepenthes (an amalgamation of the Greek *ne* meaning 'no' and *penthos* meaning 'suffering'), but what it was is anybody's guess. Homer – who refers to it in the *Odyssey* – does not explain.

Hemlock

Herbalists in ancient times also experimented with hemlock.

The Greeks gave hemlock to condemned men as capital punishment. Plato in the *Phaedo* describes how Socrates was executed with it. The executioner entered the cell carrying a cup of hemlock and explained to Socrates, 'You have nothing else to do but when you have drunk it to walk about till a heaviness takes place in your legs and afterwards lie down.' Socrates drained the cup and began walking around. He talked to his friends. Then his legs began to feel heavy, so he lay down. The executioner touched his legs from time to time, suddenly pressing hard on the toes and asking Socrates if he felt anything. Socrates said he did not.

Plato goes on: 'And Socrates also touched himself, saying that when the poison reached his heart he should then leave us. By now, his lower belly was almost cold. When uncovering himself, he said [and these were his last words]: "Crito [the name of his servant], we owe a cock to Aesculapius".' When Crito said he would see to it that the debt was paid and asked if Socrates had any other requests, there was no reply.

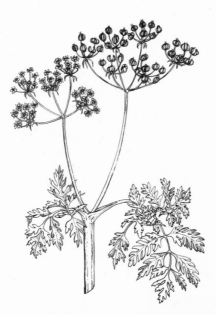

Hemlock (*Conium maculatum*)

But the herbalists found that the toxicity of hemlock varied and that it could – if prepared properly – be used to relieve pain, although the degree of relief afforded seemed to depend on the climate in which the plant grew and the age of its leaves when gathered.

The Romans used hemlock in poultices to ease sore eyes, and in the Middle Ages it was often included in 'sleeping sponges' – sponges soaked in soporific or anaesthetizing substances' which a patient sniffed before undergoing surgery. Theodoric of Cervia, author of a book on surgery in the thirteenth century, gives this recipe:

Take of opium, of the juice of the unripe mulberry, of hyoscyamus, of the juice of hemlock, of the juice of the leaves of mandragora, of the juice of the wood-ivy, of the juice of the forest mulberry, of the seeds of lettuce, of the seeds of the dock which has large round apples, and of the water hemlock: each an ounce; mix all these in a brazen vessel and then place in it a new sponge; let the whole boil, until the sponge consumes it all, and it is boiled away in it.

As oft as there shall be need of it, place the sponge in hot water for an hour, and let it be applied to the nostrils of him who is to be operated on, until he has fallen asleep, and so let surgery be performed.

But the surgeon still bound down the patient with ropes!

THE SEARCH GOES ON

The search for effective but safe pain-killers led experimenters, over the following centuries, to try some surprising things. Lady Belinda Montagu, in her book *To the Manor Born* (Gentry Books), describes this family recipe for the treatment of sciatica:

Take a pound of rosin, a pound of pitch, a pound of bees-wax. Set it on ye fire until it be melted. Then stir six peneworth of oxy-froxy. So pour it into water and oyle ye hands and work it and roll it when ye use it. Spread upon leather. It must be cut as big as yr feet and to go over yr foot. Spread very thick on ye sole of ye foot till it be on three weeks.

And this for a pain in the face: 'Thirty drops of Balsam of Peru in a glass of water. In order the better to make the balsam dissolve in the water, it should be drop'd upon a little powder of gum arabick – the Directions are, to repeat the dose in an hour if the pain does not abate.'

Belladonna, hellebore, lettuce: one by one, the herbs and flowers of the fields were tried. But because no one knew the active ingredients – what modern pharmacists call the alkaloids – only crude extracts could be made, or the whole plant used. Frequently, the result was disastrous and the patient died.

Often both doctor and patient preferred pain to death. A law was even enacted in France forbidding the use of soporific drugs before operations and the penalties were heavy; it was thought preferable to allow pain than to put life in peril.

In 1805, a young German chemist's assistant named Wilhelm

Sertürner became interested in the problem of the unreliability of drugs like opium and laudanum and decided to analyse them. Sertürner had not had a formal education but he had learned a lot from his master, and in the evenings – after the shop in Paderborn had closed – he set up his experiments.

He reasoned that there must be an active ingedient in opium – some fraction of it which could kill pain – but that the amount probably varied from plant to plant. He treated opium with water, alcohol and various other solvents and attempted to distil it. Then he had the idea of mixing it with ammonia. Sure enough, crystals were formed which had interesting properties.

He purified the crystals by washing them with sulphuric acid and alcohol, tried them on mice (which he caught in the cellar) and stray dogs (which he enticed into his back yard with titbits of meat), and dubbed his new drug 'morphium', after the God of Dreams.

He found out how much was needed to kill an animal, and then tried lesser doses on himself and his friends. In one experiment, he and three others swallowed half a grain (30 milligrammes) and then noted their reactions; swallowed another half-grain and made further notes; and took a third half-grain and attempted to record their sensations yet again, but fell over unconscious! (This is not surprising: the dose would be considered three times the maximum today.)

Sertürner continued to use morphium on himself for toothache, and it completely relieved the pain. His action in isolating the alkaloid, or active ingredient, in a natural substance won him wide acclaim, and degrees were heaped upon him by universities not only in Germany but in other countries as well, including France.

Among those who adopted Sertürner's analytical approach was a Parisian pharmacist named Henri Leroux. He was conducting experiments on willow bark, trying to isolate the active ingredient responsible for reducing fever. Eventually, in 1829, he succeeded in extracting salicin. But that is another story. . . . .

5

The Aspirin Story

Chipping Norton in the middle of the eighteenth century was a relatively bustling market town (the word 'Chipping' derives from the Anglo-Saxon 'céapari', meaning 'to cheapen', and 'Norton' means 'North town').

On the first Wednesday of each month, the pens and stalls criss-crossing the eastern slope of the town were filled with cows, sheep and pigs, and the air was thick with the cries of farmers, cheap-jacks and pedlars. The inhabitants were a mixture of rich and poor: landowners, scholars from Oxford, ladies in fine crinolines, trades-men, agricultural labourers, servants and beggars. The poor were described as 'very numerous'. The roads were rough, cows often wandered in the streets and huge trunks of timber sometimes had to be removed from the highway to allow the stagecoaches from Oxford to Birmingham through. There were about three hundred houses, mostly built of Cotswold stone, many gripped tightly by ivy. The town had a history dating back to the Roman occupation and property in many cases had been handed down from generation to generation, with family names like Tilsey, Watson and Witts perpetuating.

Every Wednesday morning, a bell would ring, signifying the opening of the market. Anybody bringing animals for sale before the bell rang was said to have 'forestalled' and was fined; indeed, in 1764 a farmer named Robinson was charged with bringing 'three couples of live fowl' nearly an hour too early. Justice was administered by a pair of constables and two assistants called 'Tything men'. Fair play in the market was ensured by two Aletasters (who checked the quality and weight of all meat, bread and beer sold) and a Leather-Sealer (who checked that all leather goods were properly tanned).

Cattle of many kinds grazed on the lush slopes of what was then common land. But moves were afoot to divide up some of the fields so that they could be more efficiently cultivated by newfangled agricultural machinery.

It was on one such Wednesday in the summer of 1758 that the Reverend Edward Stone was taking a walk on his land. He had married well – his wife (who was his stepmother's niece) hailed from a well-to-do family – and with some money from her dowry, his own savings out of the stipend of Drayton, and his dealings in Westminster, he had managed to purchase about twelve acres at Chipping Norton, adjoining the Common Brook.

He had also purchased a further two acres, nearer to the town centre, on which to reside in a 'neat commodious house' (according to a chronicler of the time),

> . . . consisting of two handsome parlours, storeroom, kitch-
> en, excellent vaulted cellars, four bedchambers and four good
> garrets, with convenient offices, brew-house, coalhouse,
> stable for five horses and dairy, with apartments over them; a
> garden and two acres of pasture adjoining, and with or without
> twelve acres of rich meadow land, at a small distance.

The 'rich meadow land' was actually rather marshy in the area of the brook, and the clergyman had to pick his way gingerly that day, in order to avoid soaking his boots and gaiters. He was fifty-six at the time and had been troubled for some years by recurrent bouts of fever, accompanied by twinges of rheumatism. He was glad not to be riding on the rough roads linking Chipping Norton with his place of work, Sir Jonathan Cope's private chapel at Bruern, eight miles away.

At the eastern corner of his meadow stood a small mill. Almost certainly, he visited it that morning on his walk. His thoughts may have been of the miller – a man named Kench who paid eighteen shillings and twopence a year for the tenancy – or of Sir Jonathan (a relative of General Sir John Cope, who had been routed by Bonny Prince Charlie at Prestonpans in Scotland thirteen years previously), or of his own son Edward, about to enter Wadham College, Oxford in his footsteps.

Whatever the object of his thoughts, he was deeply pensive as he came to a point where a footpath neatly divided his land. By that footpath stood a particularly large willow tree, its graceful fronds brushing the tips of the long meadow grasses as a breeze gently swayed it.

Almost absent-mindedly, perhaps, the clergyman plucked at a frond, stripping some of the leaves with his fingers and dirtying his hands in the process. He may have paused to cough, putting his hand to his mouth in a reflex gesture of politeness. He may have pulled out his kerchief to wipe away the crumbs of bark, then licked the fabric prior to removing the stain from his fingers. Whatever he did, *somehow* the bark reached his lips.

He was immediately struck by its bitterness. It reminded him of 'Peruvian bark', otherwise known as 'Jesuit's bark' or the bark of the South American cinchona tree (found, a century later, to be rich in quinine). Although a specific remedy for malaria (it suppresses the development of the malaria parasite), the anti-febrile action of 'Peruvian bark' had become something of a legend since it was first mentioned in European literature by Herman van der Heyden in 1643.

Could it be that the bark of this English tree – *salix alba*, or the common white willow – would react on fever and perhaps rheumaticky pain also?

The clergyman was well aware, from his study of the Humanities at Oxford, of the so-called 'Doctrines of Signatures', which implied that Nature was constantly giving signs to the observant of inner healing properties in herbs and trees, and that the best place to look for a cure was in the same geographical location as the cause – viz., the nettle and the dock leaf. Since rheumatism and certain other fevers seemed to become worse in damp conditions, was it not likely that the cure for them should be found also in damp conditions? And the willow tree loved water. He stripped off an armful of twigs and walked back to the mill.

'Here,' he told Kench the miller (or so I like to think), 'put these in a flour sack and dry them by your oven.'

During the ensuing three months, Stone delved into every book on botany he could lay hands on. Several contained references to willow bark, but there was no indication – in any which he read – of it ever having been used medicinally, although the Greek physician Dioscorides had referred to an infusion of it as 'an excellent fomentation for ye Gout'.

One day, he returned to the mill and opened the bag of twigs, which by now were crisp and baked brown from the heat of the oven. He took a knife, scraped off the bark and returned to his study, where he pulverized the flakes with pestle and mortar.

The practice of medicine at the time was still very much a matter of 'hit or miss': hospitals were virtually unheard of, most medicines were compounded from herbs by the local apothecary and bore nebulous titles such as 'Aqua Mirabilis', 'Elixir Vitae' or 'Celestial Potion', and physicians were few and far between. It was an age of self-experimentation.

I like to visualize the Reverend Edward Stone descending the stairs to his parlour one morning in cap, nightgown and blanket – cold, shivering, clearly in the grip of a fever and wondering whether he might have picked up some infectious disease. Should he try some of the brown powder in the jar over there? It might work.

I visualize him taking out a sheet of paper from his writing-desk and carefully shaking on to it enough to fill a salt-spoon, then mixing the powder with water in a goblet, quaffing the mixture and returning to bed. Four hours later, he repeated the procedure; and again, four hours after that.

By evening, his temperature had dropped. Next day he took more of the powder, gradually stepping up the dose as he felt no ill-effects. Within three days all trace of his 'ague' was gone.

'A wondrous specific, this bark,' he probably told his patron Sir Jonathan Cope at church the next Sunday, after the nobleman had enquired about his illness. 'You must allow me, sir, to treat whomsoever in your household may be unfortunate enough to submit to the ague.'

Over the next five years, the clergyman gave his powder to some fifty people, probably members of the Cope family, personal servants at Bruern and possibly friends and neighbours in Chipping Norton.

A LETTER TO THE ROYAL SOCIETY

It may have been Sir Jonathan who suggested that he should report his observations by letter to the Earl of Macclesfield, then President of the Royal Society; or it may have been Stone's own idea after reading the Society's *Philosophical Transactions* in the course of his scholastic studies. Suffice to say that by the 'two o'clock at Noon' post from Chipping Norton on 25 April 1763, the following letter was dispatched to Lord Macclesfield in the clergyman's own hand (punctuation and interpolations are mine):

My Lord,

Among the many useful discoveries which this age hath made, there are very few which better deserve the attention of the public than what I am going to lay before your Lordship.

There is a bark of an English tree which I have found by experience to be a powerful astringent, and very efficacious in curing aguish [rheumatism] and intermitting disorders [bouts of fever].

About five years ago I accidentally tasted it and was surprised by its extraordinary bitterness, which immediately raised me the suspicion of its having the properties of the Peruvian bark. As this tree delights in a moist or wet soil, where agues [rheumatic complaints] chiefly abound, the general maxim that many natural maladies carry their cures along with them, or that their remedies lie not far from their causes, was so very apposite to this particular case that I could not help applying it; and that this might be the intention of Providence here, I must own had some little weight with me.

The excessive plenty of this bark furnished me in my speculative disquisitions upon it with an argument both for and against these imaginary qualities of it; for, on one hand, as intermittents [bouts of fever] are very much common, it was reasonable to suppose that what was designed for this cure should be as common and as easy to be procured as the intermittents themselves [in other words, that a common disease should have a freely available cure]; but then, on the other hand, it seemed probable that if there was any considerable virtue in this bark it must [already] have been discovered from its plenty.

My curiosity prompted me to look into the dispensations and books of botany [existing herbal remedies] and examine what they said concerning it; but there it existed only by name. I could not find that it hath, or ever hath, any place in pharmacy, or any such qualities as I suspected ascribed to it by the botanists. However, I determined to make some experiments with it, and for this purpose I gathered that summer near a pound weight of it, which I dried in a bag upon the outside of a baker's oven for more than three months, at which time it was to be reduced to a powder by pounding and sifting, after the manner that other barks are pulverized.

It was not long before I had an opportunity of making a trial of it. But, being an entire stranger to its nature, I gave it in very small quantities – I think it was about twenty grains of the powder at a dose – and repeated it every four hours between the fits [bouts], but with great caution and the strictest attention to its effects. The fits were considerably abated, but did not entirely cease.

Not perceiving the least consequences, I grew bolder with it, and in a few days increased the dose to two scruples [20 grains or 1/24th of an ounce] and the ague was soon removed.

It was then given to several others with the same success; but I found it better answered the intention when a drachm of it [60

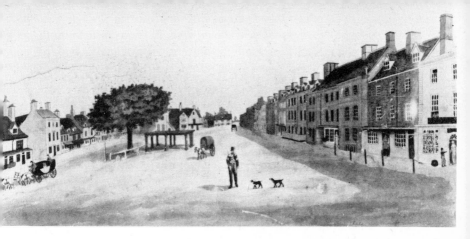

Chipping Norton in the mid–eighteenth century, when the Reverend Edward Stone lived there (PACKER'S STUDIO, CHIPPING NORTON).

Ralph Mann and the fourth-formers of Chipping Norton School stripping willow bark from a tree on what used to be the Reverend Edward Stone's land (RONALD A. STARES).

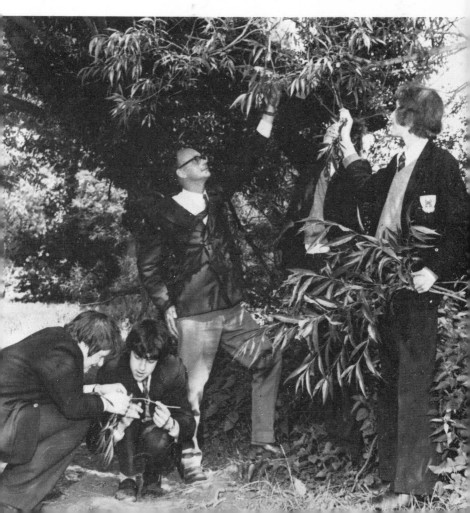

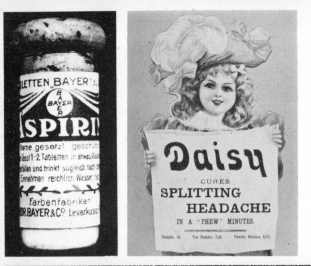

(*Far left*) An early aspirin pack (18??) of the Bayer Company (BAYER AG?)

(*Left*) Advertisement of a Victor?? patent medicine for curing headac?? (MARY EVANS PICTURE LIBRARY).

(*Below*) An opium den in the E?? End of London in Dickens's time, seen by Gustave Doré (*detail*) (MA?? EVANS PICTURE LIBRARY).

OPPOSITE PAGE
(*Above*) William Morton demonstr?? ing the first use of rectified ether o?? surgical case at Massachusetts Gene?? Hospital, 1846. (*Below*) Howev?? ether could be put to less seric?? purposes, as this 1847 illustration ?? German students getting high on ?? gas in an 'ether frolic' shows (MA?? EVANS PICTURE LIBRARY).

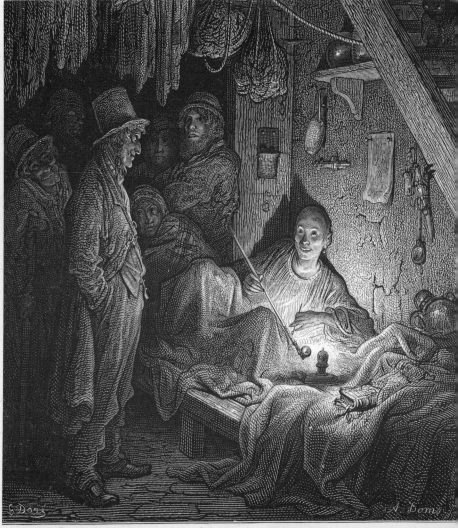

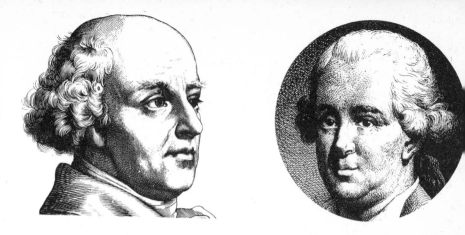

(*Above left*) Samuel Hahnemann (1755–1843), founder of the homeopathic movement (BILDARCHIV PREUSSICHER KULTURBESITZ).

(*Above right*) Franz Anton Mesmer (1733–1815). (*Below*) Mesmer's tub at his consulting room in Paris was a vat of dilute sulphuric acid, and patients sat around it either holding hands or one of the iron bars projecting from the tub (MARY EVANS PICTURE LIBRARY; ANN RONAN PICTURE LIBRARY).

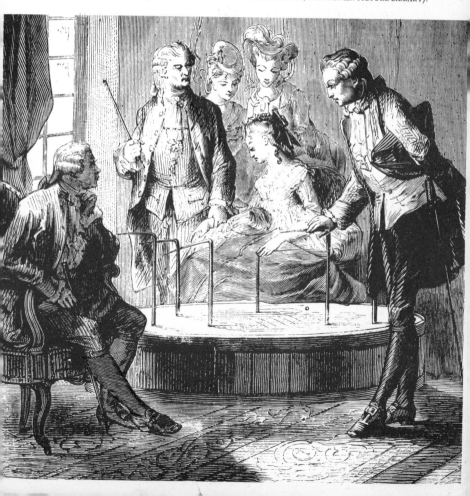

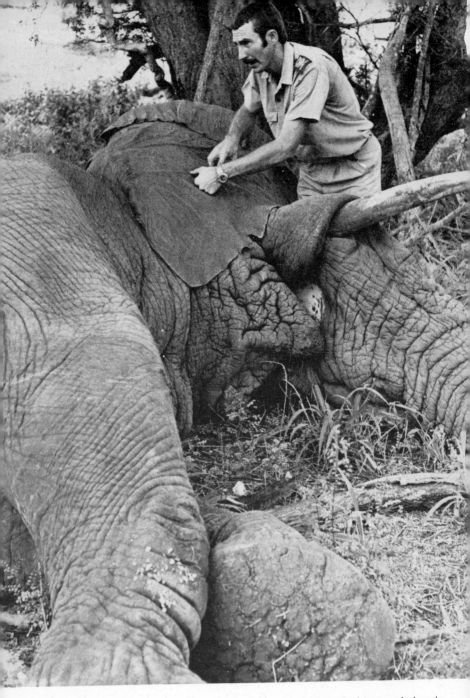

The world's most powerful knock-out drop—the drug Immobilon—fired into an elephant by a flying syringe (CAMERA PRESS).

grains or 1/8th of an ounce] was taken every four hours in the intervals of the paroxysms.

I have continued to use it as a remedy for agues and intermitting disorders for five years successively and successfully. It hath been given, I believe, to fifty persons and never failed in the cure, except in a few autumnal and quartan agues [those where the fever goes away and returns every third or fourth day] with which the patients had been long and severely afflicted. These it reduced in a great degree but did not wholly take them off; the patient, at the usual time for the return of his fit, felt some smattering of his distemper [illness] which the incessant repetition of these powders could not conquer: it seemed as if their power could reach thus far and no farther, and I did suppose that it would not have long continued to reach so far and that the distemper would have soon returned with its pristine violence, but I did not stay to see the issue. I added one-fifth part of the Peruvian bark [containing quinine] and with this small auxiliary it totally routed its adversary.

It was found necessary likewise, in one or two obstinate cases at other times of the year, to mix the same quantity of that bark with it; these were cases where the patient went abroad [got up] imprudently and caught cold, as a post-chaise boy [coach attendant] did who, being almost recovered from an inveterate tertian ague [a fever recurring every other day] would follow his business, by which means he not only neglected his powders but, meeting with bad weather, renewed his distemper.

One-fifth part was the largest – and indeed the only – proportion of the quinquina [quinine] made use of in this composition [remedy], and this only on extraordinary occasions. The patient was never prepared – either by vomiting, bleeding, purging [all treatments in use in those days] or any medicines of a similar intention – for the reception of this bark; but he entered upon it abruptly and immediately, and it was always given in powders with any common vehicles [such] as water, tea, small beer and such-like.

This was done purely to ascertain its effects, and that I might be assured the changes in the patient could not be attributed to any other thing; though, had there been a due preparation [had the medicine been made up properly] the most obstinate intermittents would probably have yielded to this bark without any foreign assistance.

By all I can judge from five years' experience of it upon a

number of persons, it appears to be a powerful absorbent, astringent, and febrifuge [anti-fever compound] in intermittent cases; of the same nature and kind with the Peruvian bark, and to have all its properties, though perhaps not always in the same degree. It seems, likewise, to have this additional quality, viz., to be a safe medicine – for I never could perceive the least ill-effects from it, though it had always been given without any preparation of the patient.

Stone's letter went on to point out that although he had taken bark from willow trees in Oxfordshire, it was probably abundant in other parts of the country. Also, the medicine might be stronger if bark from the trunk of the tree were used, instead of the branches (he had used shoots 'of three or four years growth').

He added: 'I have no other motives in publishing this specific [remedy] than that it may have a fair and full trial in all its variety and circumstances and situations, and that the world may reap the benefits accruing from it.'

But it was to be a full hundred years before the world *did* reap any further benefits from the clergyman's observations.

DETECTIVE WORK IN EUROPE

The scene shifts to Switzerland. Time moves forward half a century. In the lee of the Bernese Oberland, a Swiss pharmacist named Johann S. F. Pagenstecher is busy in his back room assembling a piece of apparatus.

There is a rat-tat-tat on the door and in troop some small children, arms piled high with wild flowers and leaves. The pharmacist points to a corner, the children stack their bundles, he gives each a small coin and they scurry away delightedly.

Pagenstecher begins to sort through the flowers, making sure they are all the same. Each plant is between three and five feet high and has tiny white flowers in a terminal cluster which give it a feathery look.

They are *Spiraea ulmaria*, otherwise known as queen-of-the-meadow or meadowsweet, and the pharmacist strips them, cascading the leaves into a vat full of water and the flowers on to the floor, where they form a thick white froth. He boils the leaves, ladling out the juice from time to time and transferring it to his apparatus, which is a form of still. The resultant clear liquid he bottles. It has a fruity smell.

Spiraea ulmaria is only one of several species of wild herb which Pagenstecher is interested in, for he is engaged on a search for substances which may help to relieve pain. He takes careful notes of each experiment and eventually sends a report of what he has observed to a Swiss scientific journal.

Pagenstecher, like many of the highly individual pharmacists of his time, was a disciple of Paracelsus, the great sixteenth-century scientist who preached the 'Doctrine of Signatures', embroidering it with the idea that each herbal remedy must contain one active ingredient put there by Nature specifically to work on one human disease. Pagenstecher, like his fellows, was trying to isolate that one active ingredient.

Whether he was aware of the therapeutic power of his little bottles of colourless liquid, we can only speculate. We assume he was. It is nice to think of villagers queuing up for their 'tincture of meadow-sweet' and then going away and applying it – either on to the skin or diluted in water – to relieve anything from gout or rheumatism to toothache or earache. The important thing was that the pharmacist's report circulated around Europe and eventually, in 1835, reached Berlin where it was read by Karl Jakob Löwig, a German chemist who was also following up the Paracelsus theory that certain plants contain an 'active' ingredient, or alkaloid.

Starting with Pagenstecher's distilled extract – known as the 'aldehyde' – he added oxygen and found that he was able to obtain an acid with quite remarkable properties. He called it 'spirsäure'. It was, in fact, salicylic acid. Thus by two different routes in three different countries, inquisitive and observant men had arrived at the basis for what was to become the world's most widely used drug. But the 'a' part of aspirin still had to be added.

In 1853, Charles Frederic Gerhardt was thirty-seven years old and Professor of Chemistry at Montpellier University. His reputation was already made. The previous year he had done some brilliant work on the preparation of acid anhydrides – substances obtained when you split up molecules of acid and remove the water – and his book *Précis de chimie organique* had become something of a best-seller in European academic circles. Gerhardt was attempting to classify organic compounds – finding out what they had in common and how they were related to each other – and amongst the substances he tackled was salicylic acid.

Salicylic acid was of considerable interest to pharmacists in those days not only because of its fever-reducing possibilities but also as a possible food preservative. Unfortunately, it was not at all palatable when swallowed. It irritated the moist membranes lining the mouth, gullet and stomach, causing actual damage if taken in quantity.

Gerhardt loved to take chemical compounds apart and put them together again in a different way, adding a little of this, taking away a little of that. When he examined the molecule of salicylic acid, he found that it comprised a central 'core' with two 'attachments': in chemical terms, a hydroxyl (OH) and a carboxyl (COOH) group of atoms extending from a six-carbon-atom benzene ring. (It was because the hydroxyl group broke away, on coming into contact with the stomach wall, that irritation was caused.)

Gerhardt decided to try a modification. He induced a reaction between acetylchloride and sodium salicylate, replacing the hydrogen atom of the hydroxyl group with an acetyl group (COCH₃). In simpler terms, he succeeded in removing a little hydrogen and substituting an ingredient of vinegar, but his procedure was so tedious and time-consuming that he rated the new substance as 'of no further significance'. And there – tantalizingly close to becoming the useful therapeutic agent which everybody was seeking – salicylic acid rested for forty years. It was used occasionally, yes. But it produced most unpleasant side-effects. Only those whose rheumatism or arthritis became intolerably painful would dare to risk its reactions.

One such person was the father of a young German chemist named Felix Hofmann. The Hofmann family lived in Elberfeld, where Felix worked for the great chemical firm of Bayer. Hofmann senior was crippled by arthritis and always in pain, except when he took a dose of sodium salicylate (a salt compounded with salicylic acid which had to be drunk in liquid form and had an unpleasant, sickly flavour).

Unfortunately, the old man had a sensitive stomach. Night after night, Felix would return home to find his father racked with pain, unable to decide which was worse – the pain of his arthritis or the pain in his gut from the salicylate. He decided to do something about it. In the Bayer laboratories he studied the process of acetylation used by Gerhardt forty years previously, and experimented until he had simplified it.

One night he took home a small phial containing his new compound, mixed it with water and gave it to his father to swallow. That night, the old man had his first pain-free sleep in years.

Felix had a colleague, Heinrich Dreser. Together they prepared experimental quantities of acetylsalicylic acid and began a programme of research to investigate how it worked in the body.

'It is self-evident', Dreser wrote, 'that only a salicylate compound which is split as soon as possible in the blood – with the liberation of salicylic acid – has medicinal value.' The acetyl part of the new formula *did* permit such a quick split.

Dreser tried it out on himself. He swallowed a solution containing one gramme of sodium acetyl salicylate and then tested his urine at intervals for twelve hours afterwards. He found traces of salicylic acid all right, but *no* trace of the sodium acetylsalicylate, which meant that the compound was breaking down beautifully in the body and liberating its 'active ingredient' into the bloodstream.

He observed that the new substance had 'a pleasant, sharp taste', as opposed to the nauseating flavour of the other medicine, and that it 'acted more gently on the walls of the stomach'.

He then wrote a scientific report recommending it for pharmaceutical use. With the agreement of the Bayer company, he and Hofmann decided to coin a name for their new drug: aspirin. 'The 'a' stood for acetyl, the 'spir' for the spiraea plant family from which the salicylic acid was obtained, and the 'in' was just there for good measure.

The year was 1899. Aspirin it was: and aspirin it has stayed ever since.

While Pagenstecher, Löwig, Gerhardt and Hofmann were pursuing their interest in meadowsweet, other chemists were investigating the properties of the willow, in parallel – but independent – lines of inquiry.

The magical power of willow leaves had been known to herbalists for a long time. Hippocrates, 2,400 years ago, had recommended a brew of them to ease childbirth. Celsus, in the first century AD, used to boil them in vinegar to treat a prolapsed uterus. Pliny recommended a paste of burnt willow bark for treating corns, and Galen used the leaves for treating bloody wounds and ulcers. In the seventeenth century, one French physician recommended them for the treatment of 'spitting of blood and all other fluxes of blood whatsoever in man or woman'.

Following publication of the Reverend Edward Stone's letter to the President of the Royal Society in 1763, willow bark was frequently prescribed for fevers, but usually as a substitute for the expensive and scarce Peruvian bark (cinchona).

An English pharmacist named White reported in 1798: 'Since the introduction of this bark into practice in the Bath City Infirmary and Dispensary, as a substitute for the Cinchona, not less than 20 pounds a year have been saved to the Charity.'

Chemists began to explore its structure, and in 1826 two Italians – Brugnatelli and Fontana – declared that the active ingredient was salicin, an extremely bitter crystalline substance with the chemical formula $C_{13}H_{18}O_7$. A Parisian, Henri Leroux, succeeded in extracting this in its pure form in 1829 by precipitating the tannin out of the bark with milk of lime, evaporating some of the residue and then dissolving out the salicin with alcohol.

A Neapolitan chemist named Raffaele Piria is credited with having been the first man to prepare salicylic acid from salicin and he did it three years after Löwig had extracted the acid from meadowsweet. Thus, by the second half of the nineteenth century, the active principle of aspirin was available from *two* sources: a tree and a flower.

A CANNY SCOT

The scene switches to Scotland, to Dundee in 1875. An amply-proportioned general practitioner in top hat and frock-coat enters a pharmacist's shop not a stone's throw from the Royal Infirmary. He is a genial man with a gentle Perthshire accent and he greets the chemist warmly, for they have done business many times: 'Morning, Mr McKay. I'd like another ounce of the white stuff,' he says, indicating two jars labelled 'Salicin'.

'Good morning, Dr MacLagan,' replies the pharmacist. 'Which one – *salix alba* or *spiraea ulmaria*?'

The doctor says he will take an ounce of each, promises to let the pharmacist know next time which he prefers, hands over four shillings and walks out. He is on his way to treat 'William R.', a 48-year-old patient with acute rheumatic fever who is not responding to conventional remedies. For four days, William R. has had a temperature around 103°F.

Over the previous week, the doctor has tried salicin on himself – first five, then ten, then thirty grains – to the great consternation of his wife, three sons and daughters. But he has felt no ill-effects.

Having studied the Humanities at Edinburgh, and read widely at the universities of Paris, Munich and Vienna, he is well aware of the 'Doctrine of Signatures' and is something of a believer in it. Furthermore, he holds the view that rheumatic fever – far from being caused by an imbalance of lactic acid, or being a disease of neurosis, as his fellow physicians suggest – is actually caused by a parasite. The parasite, he thinks, lodges in the fibrous tissue of joints, in the heart, and in muscles. Salicin, he hopes, will dislodge it.

He reaches the patient's bedside in the suburb of Dundee, examines him and leaves instructions with the mistress of the house that twelve grains of the white powder are to be given in water every three hours until the fever and temperature have subsided.

When he returns next day, he is delighted to see the patient sitting up in bed, clearly feeling much better, with temperature normal and considerably less painful swelling around his joints.

The months pass and Dr Thomas J. MacLagan tries the drug on other cases – including sufferers from rheumatism – and in each case, pain is greatly reduced. As soon as Christmas is over, he decides to prepare a paper on his use of salicin for *The Lancet*. It is published on 4 March 1876.

He wrote: 'Nature seeming to produce the remedy under climatic conditions similar to those which give rise to the disease . . . among the *Salicaceae* . . . I determined to search for a remedy for acute rheumatism. The bark of many species of willow contains a bitter principle called salicin. This principle was exactly what I wanted.'

Of his historic experiment, he wrote:

> I had at the time under my care a well-marked case of the disease which was being treated by alkalis but was not improving. I determined to give him salicin; but before doing so, took myself first five, then ten, and then thirty grains without experiencing the least inconvenience or discomfort. Satisfied as to the safety of its administration, I gave to the patient referred to twelve grains every three hours. The results exceeded my most sanguine expectations.

History was repeating itself. The drug was not, of course, killing the invading bacteria which cause rheumatic fever but *was* lessening the fever and inflammation.

Following MacLagan's report in *The Lancet*, he received a letter from a Dr Ensor who lived at the Cape of Good Hope, in which he stated that the Hottentots in Africa had for a long time used the bark of willow trees in treating rheumatic diseases. Salicin found itself in widespread demand, to the point where the price of it in the pharmacist's shop rose from two shillings to twelve shillings an ounce. Dr MacLagan went on to build up a substantial practice in London – residing at 9 Cadogan Place, SW1 – to become a Fellow of the Royal Society of Medicine and Physician-in-Ordinary to the Prince and Princess Christian of Schleswig-Holstein. Among his many rich patients were the Duchess of Albany and Thomas Carlyle.

He had the satisfaction of seeing the salicylate given a large-scale trial in at least four of the London teaching hospitals between 1877 and 1881. It became accepted as the standard treatment for rheumatic fever and, later, for gout. It was even said to be useful in diabetes.

He died on 20 March 1903 aged sixty-five, and the *British Medical Journal* gave an extraordinarily detailed account of his death:

> We regret to have to record the death on 20 March of Dr T. J. Mac-Lagan, whose writings on rheumatism in connection especially with the introduction of salicin, has made his name very familiar to the profession. Dr MacLagan had been ailing for some twelve months before his death, and by the middle of last December he had lost two

stone in weight without apparent cause. He became easily tired, and his work was carried out with difficulty. In December he began to complain of abdominal pains and of various dyspeptic troubles. Towards the end of the month a somewhat indefinite swelling was discovered in the left hypochondrium. This became more defined, and the patient became feebler and more distressed. An exploratory laparotomy was performed on 26 February. The mass was found to be part of an extensive cancerous growth of the stomach. The growth involved nearly one-half of the entire organ, and had extended to the peritoneum. No attempt at excision could be entertained, but a gastro-enterostomy was carried out. The operation relieved him of his pain, but he gradually became weaker and weaker, and sank on the morning of 20 March. He was happily spared all suffering. Through the whole of his illness he never complained, and his last concern was for the welfare of others, and not for himself. He was attended throughout the whole of his illness by Sir Thomas Barlow and Sir Frederick Treves.

The *British Medical Journal* also gave him this obituary:

Among his professional brethren, one of the first things that brought him into notice was his paper (*Lancet* Mar. 1876) on the 'Treatment of Rheumatic Fever by Salicin', published after two years' study of the properties and effects of the family of 'Salicaceae' in this disease. The reasons that led him to study this drug and eventually introduce it to the profession are interesting, because in their inception purely empirical. His observation of rheumatic fever, had impressed him with a belief that it is strongly allied to fevers of malarial or 'miasmatic' origin, and believing also that in places which seem specially favourable to the development of 'malarial' disease, Nature commonly also provides a cure, he was led to experiment with the bark of the *salix alba*, as well as with the common meadowsweet, or *spiraea ulmaria*, which also provides a salicyl compound. In 1881 he further developed his views in a monograph entitled 'Rheumatism, its Nature, Pathology and Successful Treatment' of which a second edition was published in 1896. In this he gave with much detail his reasons for rejecting the neurotic and lactic acid theories of rheumatic fever, and urged that it must be due to the life processes of a parasite having its special nidus in muscles and the fibrous tissue of the joints and heart. According to him, rheumatic fever is in essence an intermittent fever, of which the intermittences are obscured by the cycles of existence of the parasites in various foci not being coincident. In the administration of salicin he inisisted on the close repetition of large doses until pain subsided and temperature became normal.

Other works published by him were *The Germ Theory of Disease* in 1876, and *Fever: a Clinical Study* in 1888. During the last year of his life he was engaged on another book of an allied character which, though not quite completed, will, it is understood, be eventually published.

He was a Member of the Royal College of Physicians of London, and at one time on the Council of the Royal Institution, and whenever he could spare the time, took a keen and active interest in fishing and shooting.

Other doctors in other parts of Europe began to experiment with salicin. L. Reiss and S. Stricker in Berlin reported that salicylic acid was effective in treating rheumatism. Germain Sée in Paris reported that it relieved pain in arthritis and gout. And others noted that it helped with some *non*-rheumatic pains also, headache and neuralgia among them.

Meanwhile, the Bayer Company were preparing to go into mass-production of their new, pure form of acetylsalicylic acid: Aspirin. . . .

THE FIRST USE OF ASPIRIN

The first physicians to describe the medical uses of aspirin were Kurt Wilthauer and Julius Wohlgemut of Germany. Their reports, written in 1899, did not suggest that the drug had much more therapeutic effect than the old salicin derivatives, but they did point out that it was more pleasant to taste and less irritable to the lining of the patient's stomach.

A spate of similar reports followed. Migraine, persistent headache, inoperable cancer – these were just a few of the conditions said to be relieved by the new drug, which could now be made so cheaply that 'no obstacle stands in the way of its use'.

No obstacle did, at first. Hundreds of thousands of physicians in many countries began prescribing it, and in massive doses. The Bayer company – having patented all the steps in its manufacture – made a fortune. The new wonder-drug went into widespread use in Britain and in America, where in 1908 a Dr George Fetterolf gave this account of its use for the treatment of acute tonsillitis:

After the tonsils have been thoroughly cleansed, the aspirin – which should have been finely powdered in a mortar – is applied in the following manner: a small, flexible applicator is firmly but softly wrapped at the end with cotton, moistened with water, and dipped into the powdered drug. There will be found an excess of the powder gathered on the wet cotton, and this should be removed by tapping the applicator a few times. This little maneuver is quite important as otherwise, during the rubbing of the tonsil, the excess will drop off and fall into the larynx, usually causing violent paroxysms of coughing,

which on account of the inflamed condition of the throat are
exceedingly painful. With the probe thus prepared, every portion
of the tonsillar surface should be carefully and gently rubbed.

Dr Fetterolf went on:

Another method of applying the powder is by means of a
blower. I have had a large silver Eustachian catheter 'blunder-
bussed' at the end, so as to spread the powder, and use it in the
following manner: the ring end of the catheter is dipped into
the powder, which is then shaken down toward the bell-
mouthed end. After the cut-off from the compressed air-tank
has been firmly attached to the catheter, the latter is introduced
into the mouth and directed toward the tonsil. A quick jet of
air, at not over five pounds pressure, spreads the powder fairly
evenly over that portion of the tonsil toward which the catheter is pointing. This is repeated until all the available surface of
both tonsils has been covered.

Dr Fetterolf added: 'I have records of twenty-six private patients on
whom I used this method during the past year, and my results have
borne out all that is claimed for it. In all but two of the cases the relief
afforded was marked and prompt' [*The Therapeutic Gazette*, 15
November 1908].

Other American doctors began giving aspirin prophylactically –
to prevent fevers – and putting it into plasters to remove corns and
warts, while colleagues confirmed its benefits in cases of rheumatoid
arthritis, gout and rheumatic fever. It became the first line of attack
on rheumatic disease.

As Dr T. B. Begg of the Medical Research Council's Clinical
Chemotherapy Research Unit points out:

From 1876 until the present time, sodium salicylate and,
from 1899, acetylsalicylic acid (aspirin) have been the mainstay
of the chemotherapy of acute rheumatism. This is a remarkable
record. . . . Fashions in salicylate therapy have altered over the
years, and there has been frequent controversy, particularly
over the dosage and over the value of salicylate as a true cure of
rheumatic fever and as a prophylactic against the cardiac
sequelae (after-effects on the heart of rheumatic fever).

In the first few years of the twentieth century, doses of the
order of 10–13.3g (150–200 grains) per day, were being
recommended both in Britain and America, but the incidence

of side-effects with such vigorous medication was high, and more moderate doses were usually employed [A Century of Salicylates].

Assistants came and went. So did backers, despairing ever of recouping a share of the prize-money. But George persevered. Eventually, by the end of 1915, he had a sample of acetylsalicylic acid

THE BIG PRIZE

By 1914, aspirin had become so universally popular that the British Government, faced with the prospect of a total halt in supplies owing to the outbreak of hostilities with Germany, decided to launch an appeal for a 're-formulation' of aspirin, and offered a £20,000 prize to anyone in Britain or the Commonwealth who could come up with a workable, manufacturing process.

Most of the Bayer patents, which covered not only acetylsalicylic acid but many of its intermediates and also the design of manufacturing plant, still had several years to run at that time. Although the British Government was in no mood to respect commercial rights, it lacked the necessary technical information to pirate the drug on any large scale. Away from the war-zone, the United States seemed to have the appropriate background in fine chemicals but, as a non-combatant, US firms were obliged to respect the German patents.

It so happened that in Melbourne, Australia at that time there lived a chemist with considerable inventive genius and a mind set on relieving suffering. His name: George Nicholas.

Son of an enterprising Cornish miner who had emigrated after a pit disaster in 1861, George's ambition had been to become a doctor. But family penury had ruled that out. So he had turned instead to pharmacy and – at the outbreak of the First World War – had worked hard enough to become proprietor of his own corner-shop in the Melbourne suburb of Windsor. It had a low, square façade and tall Doric windows but it was what went on in the back rooms which intrigued, and then eventually concerned, neighbours.

One evening, a few months after war was declared, there was a mighty explosion and part of the roof ripped away. Windows shattered. George staggered out, hands clasped over his eyes, calling 'I can't see.' Spurred on by the £20,000 prize – to which the Australian Government had added a further £5,000 – he had been attempting to purify acetylsalicylic acid, using primitive apparatus, but a combination of heat and pressure had proved too much. A few months later, when fully recovered, he was dragged unconscious from the floor of the laboratory after being overcome by leaking gas.

pure enough to submit to the public analyst. The news got around and such interest was created that the Australian Prime Minister attended the analysis in person.

The sample passed. George Nicholas was given official permission to manufacture the acid as a 'necessary commodity'. The prize-money was his, although it took two years to materialize. There were teething troubles at first: some of the first tablets to emerge from his little 'one shot' hand-press came out pink, others yellow. But finally a product of a consistently high standard was achieved, and tests showed that it was purer even than the German tablets.

The Great War ended. As part of the price of victory, the British Custodian of Enemy Property sequested the name 'Aspirin', and the Bayer Company lost its exclusive rights to use it in Britain and in certain other countries. 'Aspirin' became a generic term for acetyl-salicylic acid and a number of pharmaceutical manufacturers moved into production of standard five-grain tablets, to British Pharmacopoeia formulation, under their own trade-names.

George Nicholas decided to call his product 'Aspro'. He had realized that with American manufacturers starting up and German aspirin beginning to come back on to the international market, he had to expand quickly – or quit. He decided on expansion. He invited his brother, Alfred, to join him in the venture (Alfred already had a successful import business). He took on more staff. He switched from packaging the tablets in sterile petrol-cans, and dispatching them via errand boys on trams, to packaging them in sterile cream tins and, finally, in so-called 'Sanitape' paper strips.

'Aspro' swept the world. It penetrated the outback (on one occasion the salesman delivered it by camel). It spread to New Zealand, Fiji and Malaya. Six years later, it entered China and then Thailand, its reputation spreading literally as fast as a sales boat called 'The Ship of Good Health' could move up the muddy waterways. Factories were set up in Asia and in Britain, as well as Melbourne; offices were opened in France, Belgium, Austria, Switzerland, Portugal, Italy and even Germany itself.

'Aspro' vans moved into Africa, showing films to villagers which spread not only the news of the fever-reducing properties of the drug but information from local government officers about vaccination as well. Hundreds of gifts of gratitude were received by the company's sales force in return, and eventually a manufacturing plant was established at Durban.

In 1926, the London firm of Gollin & Co., with offices in Mincing Lane, took a page in the 1926 *Chemist and Druggist Diary* to tell pharmacists that 'Every day is an Aspro day', promising increased turnover as a benefit of an advertised brand and proclaiming 'Aspro – Australia's biggest seller – make it yours'. The pharmacists were not impressed, however, preferring the 'generic' version. The Aspro company, determined to repeat their Australian triumph, were forced to court the grocer, and representatives actually paid the grocers' medicine licence fees to encourage them to stock their product.

However, as the numbers of people swallowing various forms of aspirin rose into the tens of millions, it became increasingly apparent that whilst the great majority could take the drug with impunity and enjoy its benefits to the full, some individuals could not.

The German physician who had first described the clinical uses of aspirin in 1899, Dr Kurt Wilthauer, had warned right from the start that tablets 'should not be swallowed whole but allowed to disintegrate first in a little sugar-water flavoured with two drops of lemon juice'. Unfortunately, many ignored his advice and swallowed crude tablets which disintegrated slowly and unevenly, bringing great lumps of acetylsalicylic acid up against the stomach wall, with damaging results. And from 1907 onwards, reports had been appearing sporadically which questioned the value of aspirin in view of its side-effects.

Research workers began to search for ways to modify aspirin so that it might be absorbed more safely. The addition of antacids was one method tried; the use of salts of aspirin – such as calcium aspirin – another.

Calcium aspirin was investigated by a number of workers who reported it to be much better tolerated than ordinary aspirin, readily soluble and more quickly absorbed into the bloodstream. In 1938 and 1939, a series of papers was published in the *British Medical Journal* and *The Lancet* which spurred the research on. In them, Dr A. H. Douthwaite, Dr G. A. M. Lintott and Sir Arthur Hurst described work they had done using a new instrument called a gastroscope. The gastroscope contained a series of lenses and mirrors, linked to a long, thin tube, which could be swallowed by the patient to show the doctor the inside of his stomach.

In one experiment, one group of patients was given a dose of ordinary aspirin and another group calcium aspirin. Some of those who took ordinary aspirin were observed to have patches of localized inflammation of the stomach-lining, whereas those who had taken calcium aspirin were normal. The inflammation was clearly seen to be a result of particles or pieces of aspirin becoming embedded in the lining, and in some cases the inflammation was sufficient to cause haemorrhage.

Dr Douthwaite was able to report that he had seen a fragment of an aspirin tablet taken by a subject, gripped in the folds of the stomach-lining, with an area of reddening denoting severe irritation of the tissue. Hurst subsequently reported the use of Douthwaite's observations in solving the problem of a man who suffered haematemesis (vomiting of blood) whilst at home, but not when in hospital. Whilst at home, it was later discovered, he swallowed aspirin tablets to which he had no access when in hospital. Examination by gastroscope after the swallowing of an ordinary aspirin tablet confirmed the cause of his complaint.

Although such extremely sensitive people seemed to be rare, the clear implication of these papers was that because many brands of aspirin tablet made at that time did not disperse in the stomach easily, and because of the slowness with which the drug dissolved in the stomach juices, it would be better if everyone could take aspirin tablets which dissolved rapidly, so that there was no risk that fragments might adhere to and irritate the stomach wall.

Calcium aspirin dissolved rapidly. But it had one major drawback: it decomposed with storage. The tablets crumbled or became soggy, liberating acetic and salicylic acid separately. Manufacturers, both large and small, were quite unable to guarantee the condition of the tablets after they left the factory; inevitably, doctors soon lost interest in this form of aspirin.

THE DISPRIN STORY

In 1938, one such small manufacturer approached the Hull-based firm of Reckitt & Colman with a sample of soluble calcium aspirin. The firm – world famous for its starch, washing 'blue' and metal polishes – had, nine years previously, moved into pharmaceutical research with a project to develop a liquid antiseptic, which would not harm the skin, and also a new disinfectant. Within four years it had perfected both: Dettol, which made a major impact on midwifery in the mid-thirties, and Sanpic, a disinfectant with a smell of fresh pine.

The research on soluble aspirin was first allotted to the company chemist, Mr Stevens, who began by examining all the products on the market containing aspirin, and in particular Alka-Seltzer. However, with the outbreak of war in 1939, Stevens joined the Armed Forces, leaving behind little of value in the way of improvement other than the addition of citric acid (to improve flavour) and a wetting agent (to prevent scumming). The project was shelved.

It so happened that working for Reckitt & Colman at that time (but on the metal polish side) was another research chemist, whose father had been a wholesale druggist and who had made him sit an examination at Leeds University in Food and Drug Analysis. His name was Harold Scruton.

With the outbreak of war, all the company's stocks of plumbago – a graphite material used in the manufacture of stove polish – were requisitioned by the Government, and Mr Scruton was given the task of re-formulating the products with alternative non-strategic materials. By 1942 he had completed the work and – with only one year left before retirement (he had joined the company in 1903) – was, in his own words, 'kicking his heels'.

One morning, the manager of the pharmaceutical department of Reckitt's, S.E. Smith, called Harold Scruton into his office and asked him if he would like to reopen the research on soluble aspirin. 'I said "yes",' Mr Scruton told me recently,

> . . . and he handed me Stevens's notes. There seemed to be two possibilities, either to pack the acetylsalicylic acid and its accompanying base separately (which would be inconvenient for the user, because he would have to mix them) or to find something which would remain stable during storage but react in water with the aspirin. It took me a year to find it.

His answer was calcium carbonate: common chalk.

Mr Scruton began by compounding his new aspirin manually, mixing the powdered chalk and salicylic acid in a tin and then tamping the mix into small, round tablets using a punch and die.

'But the first ones simply dropped to the bottom of the glass,' he recalls. 'Nothing happened. No reaction. Nothing. It was very disappointing.'

By a curious quirk of fate, all Mr Scruton's work was having to be carried out on the scrubbed tables of Reckitt & Colman's large laundry because German bombers had devastated his laboratory (and much of the remainder of the works in Dansom Lane, Hull) in a raid on 19 July 1941. Looking around, while his tablets rested recalcitrantly on the bottom of the glass, his eye alighted on a packet of the company's starch: 'It suddenly occurred to me that starch, too, was insoluble and therefore should be stable, but it might be just the thing to get the reaction going in the water. It was ironical that it was the Germans, in a roundabout way, who led me to the answer.'

He tamped together a fresh mix. To his delight it worked: the aspirin in the tablets dissolved within seconds.

'By adding the starch, I not only got a reaction but the starch actually allowed the water to penetrate the salicylic acid better,' he went on. 'Mind you, we found by experimentation that there had to be an ideal quantity: too much starch made the tablet difficult to compress and also to transport; it fell to bits if it got knocked about.'

About 300 further experiments were conducted, and more than 1,000 analyses. Finally, Harold Scruton was satisfied with what he nicknamed 'Sol-prin', and the project was turned over to one of the company engineers, Mr F. A. Parish, to make the equipment needed for mass-production of calcium aspirin.

Mr Colman Green, who became Head of Pharmaceutical Research at Reckitt & Colman takes up the story:

So far as he was able to develop them at all during wartime, Mr Scruton's mechanical problems were no less formidable than his chemical problems. In the earliest stages of his work, he needed a means of producing a few tablets quickly to ascertain whether a particular experimental mixture produced tablets at all, and, if it did, to produce the tablets to put on test.

His tablet-making equipment is well remembered by the few members of the laboratory staff who remained at Dansom Lane during the war years. Mr H. L. Coulson recalls – now with some degree of nostalgia – the characteristic series of noises emanating from the bench at which Mr Scruton was hammering out experimental tablets.

First, he recalls the characteristic noise of the powder-mixing operation – rolling a lever-lid tin on its side along the bench-top, from one end to the other and back again, repeating the motion as often as necessary. The swish of the tin contents, as it mixed in the rolling tin, the metallic noise as the tin rolled over unevennesses in the bench top, all accompanied by the sound of Mr Scruton's measured tread as he walked the tin backwards and forwards along the bench on its purposeful journey, were part of the sound scene.

Then – less tolerable – was the characteristic noise emanating from the punching of the tablet from the mixed powders. All one required was, as it were, three pieces of steel and a hammer. There was a heavy sheet-steel bed-plate, on which stood a heavy mild steel die; and, finally, a punch. This equipment reduced tablet-making to its basic operations and is worth considering carefully because our modern 32-punch high-speed tabletting machines work exactly on the same basic principle.

The periodical 'rat-tat-tat-TAT', followed presumably by the hammer being dropped on the bench in the approved manner, led to much jangling of the nerves of colleagues endeavouring to concentrate on their own stress-provoking problems in this open laboratory.

Before he retired, however, Mr Scruton saw the arrival of an electrically-driven rotary press, capable of making sixteen tablets simultaneously, and was told by the company that the new product would be marketed under the trade name 'Disprin'.

'I think', he recalled thirty years later when I interviewed him in his home, 'that this project gave me more satisfaction than anything else I have ever done.'

Clinical trials at a London teaching hospital confirmed that the new tablet possessed all the therapeutic properties of calcium aspirin; tests in the Reckitt & Colman laboratories confirmed that it was stable when mass-produced, and suitable for tropical – as well as temperate – climates. But there were manufacturing problems. Once again, Mr Colman Green explains:

> I was now confronted with the dilemma that whilst Mr Scruton's unorthodox formulation just could not be altered, it did not seem likely that conventional tabletting plant and processes could produce tablets from it.
>
> Mr Scruton went about it with an ingenious but primitive bench-top unit. He weighed the mixed powders into the die before compacting them. This would not be practicable in mass-production. The powder has to be measured *volumetrically*, which means two important requirements: first, its bulk density must be constant (or very nearly so); second, the powder must be in a form capable of *flowing* into a die. It is a matter of common experience that, for example, sugar will flow freely from a bag, but flour will not. So the 'Disprin' mixed powders, which are rather like flour, have to be treated in some way to enable them to flow rather like sugar. This is done by a process called 'slugging', by which the powder is highly compressed into a very large 'slug' (which is really a very large cylindrical tablet) in a highly controlled way. This slug is then 'kibbled' (broken up) into largish particles and sieved. The resulting powder will now flow freely, smoothly and rapidly into the dies of a rotary tablet-machine from a hopper.
>
> So we had to find the required items of plant. But where? 'Up to five years' was the delivery-period quoted by plant manufacturers: we had to extemporize.

Presses which had survived the Blitz that had been used in the manufacture of Reckitt's Blue and Reckitt's Bath Cubes, proved incapable of being adapted to our requirements. Fortunately, the engineering department were able to locate some single-punch presses which were surplus to requirements in a Government explosives factory. Belt-driven, they had to be set up for trial in the only place with a belt-drive – in the engineering shop itself; and there, at some hazard to body and limb on its temporary bed, some slugs were turned out after substantial rebuilding of the machines.

The mixing of the powders was tricky, and here again delivery of suitable mixers was very prolonged. So one had to be built in the engineering shop. It so happens that as a member of one of the British Industrial Objectives Survey export teams operating in the American and French Army Zones, and following the fighting forces as they penetrated into Germany in the summer of 1945 in order to uncover scientific and industrial war secrets, I had come across a simple, but ingenious, batch mixer, easily capable of being built in our own shops. This course was adopted and these mixers have given excellent results over the decades ever since.

'Disprin' was launched on the medical profession in 1948 at the London Medical Exhibition. Mr Colman Green recalls:

I clearly remember the enthusiastic interest of the doctors who literally thronged the stand to hear about 'Disprin'. There was a continual flow of complimentary remarks in which such phrases constantly appeared as: 'Just what was wanted'; or 'Just what we have all been waiting for'. Success now stared us in the face!

Our new analgesic preparation 'went like a bomb'. But this quickly put us in the real trouble which I had so feared. The increasing demand for 'Disprin' soon exceeded the capacity of the original pilot-plant by a large margin. The only way to meet demand was to work two shifts.

The primary bottle-neck was the capacity of the air-conditioning plant, which now became heavily overloaded by the moisture arising from the increasing number of 'bods' working in the room. At times, especially when the outside conditions were humid, people had to be withdrawn from the room temporarily until the conditioner was able to bring the atmosphere into control again. This procedure had to be constantly repeated during the shifts.

The arrangements, which were tedious and harassing for all concerned, continued for months, until the new and enlarged plant which had been so long on order, arrived and was installed.

Soon, reports were flowing in indicating that the new soluble tablets were better tolerated than ordinary aspirin, especially by those who required large doses over long periods. Independent tests carried out in another London hospital showed that Disprin allowed aspirin to be absorbed more rapidly into the blood, and confirmed its ability to produce the requisite level of salicylate in the bloodstream necessary for the treatment of certain rheumatic disorders.

In 1951, Reckitt & Colman decided to prepare a soluble aspirin especially for prescription under the National Health Service; ironically, they chose the name which Harold Scruton had originally given to his formulation 'Solprin'.

Disprin and Solprin quickly gained wide acceptance amongst medical practitioners. In 1952, a monograph published in the *British Pharmacopoeia* gave official recognition to the contribution made by the former to salicylate therapy. But by that time the public had shown its own approval, thanks partly to a clever series of advertisements which appeared in 1949–50 with the slogan 'Take an aspirin – I mean a Disprin'.

In 1955, a quarter-strength tablet – Disprin Junior – was launched, to save parents the trouble of breaking their tablets into pieces. Each tablet was individually wrapped in foil, thereby minimizing the chances of a child gaining access to more than one tablet at a time. In 1974, Disprin was re-formulated. Most of its original starch was removed, thus making it dissolve more completely and more rapidly. Whereas the original drug would dissolve in cold water in thirty-seven seconds, the new formulation dissolved in fifteen. Sales boomed.

ASPIRIN TODAY

Disprin apart, the *British Pharmacopoeia* lists scores of preparations containing aspirin, and by 1973 had published five monographs: 'Aspirin', 'Aspirin Tablets', 'Soluble Aspirin Tablets', 'Aspirin Phenacetin and Codeine Tablets' and 'Soluble Aspirin, Phenacetin and Codeine Tablets'. Subsequently, three amendments have appeared: 'Aspirin and Codeine Tablets', 'Soluble Aspirin and Codeine Tablets' (the last two after the withdrawal of Phenacetin from preparations) and finally, 'Aspirin and Caffeine Tablets'.

Aspirin has become the most widely used – and probably the most trusted – drug in the world today. Hundreds of millions of people swallow it each year. In America, more than 6,500 tons of aspirin are sold annually, while in Britain something like 4,000 million tablets are consumed by the public each year.

Thousands of experiments have been carried out with aspirin, in hospitals and laboratories. Dozens of alternative substances have been examined, and found wanting. It has been taken to the bottom of the oceans, up Everest, and even to the moon and back. And yet nobody is sure precisely how it works. . . .

Aspirin is a three-in-one – some say a four-in-one – drug. It brings down fever; it reduces inflammation; it deadens pain. But it also alters the coagulation potential of blood, so that some doctors recommend a regular dose of aspirin to avoid the risk of a heart attack (indeed, one form of aspirin is sold in Germany specifically for that purpose).

Furthermore, unlike most other pain-killers, it often sounds an alarm-bell – literally – if the user takes too much. It produces a ringing in the ears – known as tinnitus – when too high a dose is swallowed.

The drug begins life in the laboratory as salicylic acid, which is obtained by modifying the so-called 'benzene ring', the basic structure of thousands of organic chemicals. Another chemical structure known as the 'acetyl group' (of atoms) is then tagged on to this to produce acetylsalicylic acid. (The acetyl group is also present in acetic acid and gives vinegar its tangy smell.)

It is absorbed fairly rapidly into the bloodstream through the wall of the stomach or – even more rapidly – through the upper intestine. The maximum level of acetylsalicylic acid is reached in the blood and tissues after about two hours, and in only thirty minutes in the case of soluble aspirin. (Slightly different absorption rates are achieved with different forms of aspirin.)

Once inside the body, some of the aspirin molecule is broken down into salicylate, which in turn is broken down into a variety of other substances. It spreads evenly around the body, also penetrating the brain, where some of its most useful work is done.

Traces of a single aspirin tablet can be detected in the body as long as seventy-two hours later, although most of the drug is excreted within fifty hours. Excretion is handled by the kidneys and leaves the body mainly in the urine.

The active ingredient has an effect on many of the chemical processes which occur in the body: it alters metabolism in several ways. Firstly, it steps up the body's consumption of oxygen (by acting on enzymes). Secondly, it affects the way the body handles carbohydrates (starch, sugar, and so forth). Thirdly, it lowers levels of fats in the blood when given in large doses. Fourthly, it affects the clotting mechanism of blood. Fifthly – again when given in large doses – it will lower the amount of uric acid in the blood. And finally, it affects the body's nitrogen balance. Such versatility means that it can be used for the treatment of a whole range of diseases.

Fevers. Human body temperature is regulated from a region of the brain known as the hypothalamus. Aspirin has no effect on the hypothalamus if the temperature is normal. But if it is raised – in other words, if the person has a fever – then the aspirin persuades the hypothalamus to dilate blood-vessels in the skin, all over the body. Heat is then lost, both by radiation and through sweating. It is, in fact, a thermostat.

Although the first widespread use of aspirin was on rheumatic fever, all fevers have since been found to respond to the drug, in that the patient's temperature is lowered.

Inflammation. When a part of the body becomes inflamed, blood-vessels in the area dilate. Fluid seeps out of the bloodstream and into the tissues. The area swells and grows red. The patient feels a 'hot spot' and pain. Aspirin suppresses the inflammatory process, but exactly how, nobody is yet sure. It quickly removes the collection of fluid from tissues and causes inflamed joints to shrink back in size, but whether this is done by some local action on the blood-vessels or by a more roundabout mechanism is still not completely explained.

Pain relief. Millions of people know that aspirin reduces pain, but for years scientists had difficulty proving it. Then James Hardy, Harold Wolff and Helen Goodell of Cornell University invented their 'dolorimeter' and were able to show – by focusing a beam of heat on the forehead of volunteers who had swallowed aspirin – that it definitely did deaden pain and that the maximum effect was obtained by taking two tablets (600 milligrammes). They also observed that the drug was excellent for 'moderate' pain but brought little or no relief in cases of sudden injury or stomach pains.

Later, Lt-Col Henry Beecher – who carried out the original work on attitudes to pain at the Anzio beachhead – demonstrated on hospital patients that two aspirin tablets produced the same amount of relief as an injection of ten milligrammes of morphine; in other words, aspirin is about one fiftieth as analgesic as morphine.

But how does it act?

At first, researchers suggested that it might exert its influence solely on the brain; then others claimed that it acted locally, on nerves in the area where the pain was felt. Today, it is believed to act on both. Unquestionably, it will relieve a whole variety of pains: toothache, most headaches, lumbago, period pains, tonsillitis and rheumatic pain amongst them. And people who gargle with it swear that it has an analgesic effect on a sore throat, which certainly (since they do not swallow it) bears out the impression that it has some local action.

Much research is now being carried out into the action of aspirin in the body, if for no other reason than that an explanation may throw light on the mechanism of a number of other substances and several diseases.

It has been suggested that one of its actions is against the natural peptides called kinins. K. S. Lin and colleagues at the Miles Laboratories carried out a series of experiments in the early 1960s which showed that aspirin blocked the action of one – bradykinin – and suppressed excitation of nerve-endings in the viscera which promote the sensation of pain. But not all types of pain produced by bradykinin were blocked, nor was it established that it blocked bradykinin-induced pain any better than sensations from other painful stimuli.

Researchers next turned their sights on the mechanism by which the bronchioles of guinea-pigs could be made to constrict in mimicry of human asthma. Two substances released during anaphylactic shock were found to be capable of doing this, one known simply as SRS-A (for Slow Reacting Substance in Anaphylaxis), the other the family group of kinins. But the action of both could be completely prevented by administration of a small dose of aspirin a few minutes before the injection.

H. O. J. Collier, in 1963, reported:

Although aspirin has no such effect on the action of histamine, it appears to act as a specific chemical antagonist of kinins and SRS-A, just as antihistamines antagonize histamine. If the three substances are jointly responsible for the bronchospasm, one might expect that treatment with both aspirin and antihistamine would prevent it and that either drug would be partly effective.

Within the past year, Alexander R. Hammond, Barbara Whiteley and I have found strong evidence in support of this prediction. In this particular model of asthma, at least, it appears that aspirin acts as a pharmacological antagonist of kinins and SRS-A. This effect is probably achieved by the molecules of aspirin blocking a reaction between the molecules of kinins, SRS-A and the bronchial muscle they stimulate.

He continued:

From clinical experience it is known that aspirin and antihis-tamines, when taken separately, ameliorate asthma slightly in human patients. But it is not yet established that the two drugs, taken together, would have a stronger effect, or that aspirin acts as a pharmacological antagonist of kinins or SRS-A in the human lung [*Scientific American*, no.209, 1963].

As far as its anti-inflammatory action is concerned, researchers have tried to show that aspirin may act by stimulating production of steroids from the adrenal glands.

In the early 1960s, B. B. Newbould of Imperial Chemical Industries found that acetylsalicylic acid, sodium salicylate, phenylbutazone, aminopyrine and flufenamic acid, the most effective types of non-steroidal agents in the treatment of human rheumatoid arthritis, showed corresponding potencies when administered to rats. Newbould's research indicated that among drugs known to be effective against the human disease, only the quinoline antimalarials were ineffective against the rat arthritis. His experiments affirmed the similarity between the laboratory model of arthritis and the human disease, and demonstrated the powerful anti-inflammatory action of aspirin and related drugs.

Other research has shown that large doses of aspirin can stimulate the adrenals and produce side-effects typical of steroid therapy ('moon-facing' etc.); but similar side-effects have been demonstrated in animals with no adrenals and in humans whose adrenal glands have been destroyed by disease.

The drug definitely has an effect on antigen-antibody reactions and can exert a modulating effect on the thyroid gland.

The latest theory is that aspirin may produce *all* its effects – pain-killing, temperature lowering and anti-inflammatory – by blocking production of prostaglandins (hormone-like substances which play a key role in regulating cell-metabolism). It is this possibility which has excited a fresh burst of enthusiastic experimentation, for prostaglandins have become the 'queen substance' of modern pharmaceutical research.

Early evidence of this came from J. R. Vane, then of the Pharmacology Department of the Royal College of Surgeons, when he reported (in June 1971) results of his experiments on lung tissue taken from guinea-pigs:

'Prostaglandin release can often be equated with prostaglandin synthesis,' he explained (*Nature New Biology*, vol. 231), 'for many tissues can be provoked to release more prostaglandin than they contain. The possibility arises, therefore, that anti-inflammatory substances such as aspirin inhibit the enzyme(s) which generate prostaglandins. The experiments described below were designed to test this possibility.'

At the end of his tests, Vane concluded: 'Aspirin . . . strongly inhibits prostaglandin synthesis. This may be the mechanism underlying its therapeutic action.'

In the same journal, J. B. Smith and A. L. Willis reported how aspirin selectively inhibited production of prostaglandin in human platelets. They concluded:

> Aspirin administered inhibited the production of prostaglandins in the platelet in a system in which 'the release reaction' was unimpaired. . . . Aspirin inhibits 'the release reaction' when induced by collagen or low concentrations of thrombin. In our experiments, relatively high concentrations of thrombin (5 U/ml.) were used and as a result aspirin did not inhibit the release of the platelet constituents. The production of prostaglandins is thus dissociated from 'the release reaction'. The finding that the production of prostaglandins is inhibited by aspirin, while the release of phospholipase A is unaffected, strongly suggests that one action of aspirin on platelets is inhibition of the conversion of arachidonic acid into prostaglandins. Other work from this laboratory has shown that aspirin inhibits the synthesis of prostaglandins from arachidonic acid in guinea-pig lung homogenates. . . .

They added, 'If the prostaglandins are indeed important mediators of inflammation, the clinical effectiveness of aspirin and indomethacin as anti-inflammatory agents could be explained by the inhibition of the production of prostaglandins.'

In 1972, Dr Charles de Witt Roberts reported in *The Lancet* (13 May, p.1070) how he had found, by statistical analysis, that aspirin reduced the concentration of Prostaglandins E and F in samples of seminal fluid. Commenting on this a few months later, Dr E.R. Trethewie of the Department of Physiology at the University of Melbourne wrote:

> This mechanism is in accord with the effects of acetylsalicylic acid. This acid inhibits the release of histamine and S.R.S. (Slow Reacting Substance) – once thought to be prostaglandin – in the antigen/antibody reaction of anaphylaxis. I believe that aspirin inhibits the release of these substances by interfering with antibody groupings. Further, I have shown that aspirin also reduces the output of histamine in venom injury and that blood – probably its protein constituents – plays an essential part in the reaction. It is possible that aspirin interferes with a membrane lipoprotein precursor releasing prostaglandin E and F.

Summing up the situation in a leading article (5 May 1973), *The Lancet* confirmed:

> It is reasonable to propose that the anti-inflammatory activity of drugs such as aspirin, indomethacin, and phenylbutazone may be due, at least in part, to blockade of prostaglandin synthesis. The antipyretic actions of these drugs could be explained on the same basis, since some prostaglandins are potent pyrogens. It has also been suggested

that inhibition of prostaglandin synthesis could account for the gastro-intestinal toxicity of anti-inflammatory drugs and that aspirin might prevent abortion and interfere with the function of intra-uterine contraceptive devices. Thus, many of the actions of aspirin-like drugs could be explained by a common mechanism.

The leader went on:

Until lately, analgesia – one of the most important actions of aspirin – could not be clearly related to effects on prostaglandins. Attempts to produce pain by injection or application of prostaglandins have yielded conflicting results, and as much as 100 milligrammes per millilitre of prostaglandin E2 on a blister-base produced no pain. Grylglewski and Vane have proposed that the pain of inflammation is produced by an unstable cyclic peroxide intermediate in the biosyn-thesis of prostaglandins, and there is evidence that this precursor is the mysterious rabbit-aorta-contracting substance (R.C.S.). Aspirin-like drugs prevent the release of R.C.S., a bronchoconstrictor produced in the lungs of sensitized guinea-pigs. Ferreira has now produced further evidence in support of the hypothesis that pain can be caused by lipoperoxides and prostaglandins. He compared the pain-producing activity of fatty-acid hydroperoxides, acetylcholine, bradykinin, histamine, and prostaglandin E1 after intradermal injection and sub-dermal infusion in volunteers. The fatty-acid hydroperoxides were prepared by incubating linoleic, linolenic, and arachidonic acids with lipoxidase, and they caused intense but short-lasting pain accom-panied by a mild erythema. These effects were not produced by the parent fatty acids. Acetylcholine, histamine, and bradykinin pro-duced pain which disappeared within five minutes, but prostaglandin E1 caused strong pain and hyperalgesia which lasted for up to four hours. Slow subdermal infusions of prostaglandin E1 in concentra-tions of the same order as those found in inflammation caused hyperalgesia, a sensitization to chemical or mechanical stimuli which is a characteristic of all types of inflammation. This effect was depen-dent on the concentration infused and the duration of infusion, sug-gesting that the continued release of minute amounts of prostaglandin at a site of injury will gradually produce a hyperalgesic state, perhaps by sensitizing pain receptors.

These observations show that lipoperoxides and prostaglandins can cause overt pain, depending on their concentrations, but in inflammatory reactions they probably only sensitize receptors to pain. Aspirin-like drugs can inhibit the synthesis of lipoperoxides as well as prostaglandins, and their analgesic action may after all be explained by this mechanism.

In 1977, John Vane (who had become Director of Group Research and Development at the Wellcome Foundation) received $15,000 and the Albert Lasker Medical Research Award for his work on prostaglandins and particularly for his role in the isolation of prostacyclin – the substance whose major action is now known to be the prevention of the formation of blood clots such as those which lead to heart attacks and strokes. The citation stated:

> Dr Vane and his colleagues have shown that the walls of blood-vessels produce prostacyclin, which prevents platelets from clumping. Another significant milestone was Dr Vane's discovery that aspirin-like drugs inhibit the formation of prostaglandins. He proved that this action is the basic mechanism of the therapeutic effect, a theory now widely accepted.
>
> Dr Vane devised a simple method for the bioassay of prostaglandins which he and his colleagues have used over the years. This has resulted in a new body of knowledge about the role which prostaglandins play in health and disease.

But there are still things to learn about aspirin, and the research goes on. For the moment, the matter may be left in the words of H. O. J. Collier:

> Whether aspirin, in its vast consumption, is taken as an antipyretic, analgesic or antirheumatic, its general function seems to be the moderation of the defensive reactions to various forms of disease. It would appear that the human body has an unwieldy defence establishment that aspirin fortunately can help to control.

So much for *how* aspirin works. But why has it become the world's most widely consumed drug?

On Friday, 30 May 1975 an 'Aspirin Symposium' was held at the Royal College of Surgeons in London. The first speaker – Dr Gordon Fryers of Reckitt & Colman, London – pointed out that an estimated 35,000 tons of aspirin was being consumed throughout the world each year, 1,500 tons of it in Britain. That was equivalent to forty-five doses of two tablets for every man, woman and child. The cost worked out at less than thirty pence per year.

Referring to aspirin's effect on body temperature – bringing it down when raised but not influencing it when normal – Dr Fryer added: 'Doctors have long felt that a medicine that regulated the abnormal but did not interfere with the normal was hopelessly Utopian. Perhaps aspirin is a step in this direction and perhaps this explains why it is such a good home medicine.'

Headaches (of which 5,000,000 are estimated to occur each day in Britain alone), colds, influenza, most fevers, and pain of a great variety of kinds: all these have become standard recipients of treatment by aspirin. In 1971, the council on drugs of the American Medical Association described aspirin as the 'drug of choice' when a mild analgesic or antipyretic was indicated, and the 'primary agent' used in the management of some rheumatic diseases. Aspirin, said the council, is

> . . . more useful in treatment of headache, neuralgia, myalgia, arthralgias, and other pains arising from integumental structures than in acute pain of visceral origin, but may be effective in less severe postoperative and postpartum pain or in pain secondary to trauma and cancer. In the latter, aspirin may provide adequate relief and should be tried prior to use of more potent drugs. . . . When drug therapy is indicated for reduction of fever, aspirin is one of the most effective and safest drugs.

At the 1975 'Aspirin Symposium', details were given of the use of aspirin for treating various rheumatic diseases and pain in cancer.

First, Dr F. Dudley Hart, consultant in rheumatic disorders at the Westminster Hospital, reported:

> In the now comparatively-rare disease of rheumatic fever, salicylates are still first choice. . . .
>
> Aspirin is useful in easing pain arising from bursitis, periarthritis and a host of other extra-articular, non-arthritic conditions. It does not, however, affect the natural history of these disorders, which take their own time to get better. . . .
>
> Aspirin can be given occasionally to relieve the pain of rheumatoid arthritis or at regular intervals throughout twenty-four hours as an anti-inflammatory agent. . . . With doses of around five grammes daily there is considerable reduction of swelling within a few days [but] to get five grammes daily of aspirin in to a patient is not always easy. . . .
>
> Aspirin is helpful in both varieties of osteo-arthritis . . . relief usually commences in fifteen to thirty minutes but seldom lasts longer than two to four hours.

However, Dr Dudley Hart reported that aspirin had not proved of great practical value in the treatment of acute gout. 'While it can ease the pain in mild attacks,' he added, 'it does not control the symptoms of severe, acute gout nearly as well as other agents.'

His observations made an interesting comparison with comments made by the American Rheumatism Association in its *Primer on the Rheumatic Diseases*, issued eleven years previously, from which the following extracts are taken:

1. *Rheumatoid arthritis*. In a considerable proportion of patients, aspirin is the only drug needed . . . its capacity to suppress the symptoms and often the signs of chronic inflammatory articular disease is extraordinary and is usually clearly recognized by the patient himself.
2. *Ankylosing spondylitis*. Full and regular doses of salicylates constitute a critical part of the program, and, combined with physical therapy, may prove sufficient.
3. *Fibrositis*. If any relief at all is achieved with salicylates, full and regular doses should be employed.
4. *Rheumatic fever*. Most authorities now treat rheumatic fever with salicylates, rather than corticosteroids, when no evidence of carditis exists. . . . Salicylates are usually given as aspirin.
5. *Degenerative joint disease (osteo-arthritis, osteo-arthrosis)*. Salicylates, particularly aspirin, in moderate doses are usually helpful and, in combination with rest and physical measures, constitute adequate drug therapy in most cases.

Aspirin's role in suppressing pain in cancer patients was described at the symposium by Stanley Wallenstein of the Sloan-Kettering Institute for Cancer Research, New York. He reported that aspirin, in doses of five grammes, had proved 'effective in relieving mild to moderate pain in patients with cancer for periods of up to six hours'.

'Although responses of individual patients vary,' he went on, 'studies in relatively small groups of patients have been able to discriminate between the analgesic effects of aspirin and placebo, as well as between graded doses of aspirin.' He concluded: 'Combinations of aspirin with narcotics, such as morphine and codeine, produced additive analgesic effects, suggesting that these drugs act by different mechanisms and that there is a real clinical advantage in administering them together.'

But an even more potentially valuable role for aspirin was indicated at the same symposium: as a weapon, in the future, against heart disease. Because doctors had noticed that the blood of people taking regular doses of aspirin became less 'sticky' than usual, scientists had examined its action on tiny components in the blood known as platelets. Dr P. C. Elwood, Director of the Medical Research Council's Epidemiology Unit at Cardiff, summed up the situation like this:

There is growing evidence that platelet aggregation is a major factor in arterial thrombosis and that platelets may be involved in atherosclerosis. There is, therefore, great interest in drugs which affect platelet function, as these may modify the course of cardiovascular disease. Interest arises at two levels. Firstly, present knowledge of aetiological mechanisms involved in cardiovascular disease is grossly deficient, and if an alteration in some aspect of platelet function were shown to affect some manifestation of cardiovascular disease, a relevant mechanism would have been identified and further research facilitated. Secondly, whatever the mechanisms involved, a drug which may reduce the incidence of one of the most important causes of death will naturally arouse very great interest.

Dr Elwood went on:

There are several drugs which modify platelet function, but the one on which greatest attention is focused at present is aspirin. Evidence from 'test-tube' and observational studies is suggestive but there is no conclusive clinical evidence of benefit. A large randomized controlled trial of aspirin in the prevention of death in men who had had a myocardial infarct has been described (*British Medical Journal* 1974, vol. 1, no. 436). The results of this trial are suggestive but not conclusive. But further trials are in progress in this and in other countries. If benefit is confirmed, there will be important implications for prophylaxis and for research.

Prophylaxis? Could it be that we shall one day see aspirin taken on a widespread scale to ward off cardiovascular disease, the number one killer in the Western world? Actually, the idea is not new.

Dr Len Wood of the City of Hope Medical Centre, California, wrote in *The Lancet* as long ago as 9 September 1972:

I suggest that men over the age of twenty and women over the age of forty should take one aspirin tablet (0.325 g) a day on a chronic, long-term basis in the hope that this will lessen the severity of arterial thrombosis and atherosclerosis. Exceptions to this would be people with bleeding disorders, aspirin allergy, uncontrolled hypertension, and those with a history of bleeding lesions of the gastro-intestinal tract or other organ system.

Further evidence of the drug's value in the treatment of heart disease was given in 1972, when Dr Jeffrey Frank of New Jersey College and his brother Dr Nathan Frank of Georgetown University, Washington reported (*Annals of Internal Medicine*, vol. 78, no.3):

We have used this therapy, usually 600 mg of aspirin daily, for approximately four years and have been impressed with the results. We realize that ours is simply a clinical impression, but logic and the present evidence of the mechanism of thrombogenesis indicate that this treatment has substance.

If our impression is substantially corroborated, we propose that all middle-aged persons take 600 mg of aspirin daily. Let us do something to reduce the incidence of coronary-artery occlusive disease.

There is an indirect means that may help convince competent cardiac investigators that aspirin therapy is worthy for treatment of patients with potential or established ischemic heart disease due to coronary-artery disease.

We suggest a study on this basis. It is generally recognized that the incidence of coronary-artery disease and acute myocardial infarction is low in patients with rheumatoid arthritis; the reason has been unknown. The basic drug used by patients who have had this disease for many years is aspirin, in spite of the advent of many other drugs, such as adrenal cortico-steroids, phenylbutazone and gold. We propose a survey of the necropsy findings and clinical histories for coronary-artery disease and myocardial infarction in those patients who have been taking aspirin for many years.

Shortly after this article appeared, a proper study of the use of aspirin in preventing secondary infarcts in people who had survived one heart attack was set up in America. Called the 'Coronary Drug Project Aspirin Study' (CDPA) it involved 1,529 patients attending 53 clinical centres – 758 patients being given one 324 mg aspirin tablet three times a day, and 771 patients being given a placebo, or dummy, tablet (see figure). When the trial ended in February 1975, the death-toll amongst the aspirin-takers was only 5.8 per cent, compared to 8.3 per cent in the placebo group – a reduction of 30 per cent! The number of patients involved in this first survey was, of course, small. But the results were sufficiently encouraging to warrant the launching of two much larger research projects which, at the time of writing, are still running.

One is the 'Aspirin Myocardial Infarction Study' (AMIS) in which 4,524 patients are taking part – all of whom have suffered one heart attack. A total of 2,267 are being given one 500 mg aspirin capsule twice daily, while 2,257 are being given a placebo.

The other is the 'Persantine-Aspirin Reinfarction Study' (PARIS) in which 2,026 patients are taking part. In this trial, the drug in use is aspirin combined with Persantine (dipyridamole), a product of the Boehringer-Ingelheim pharmaceutical company: 810 patients are being given aspirin alone, 810 aspirin plus Persantine, and 406 a

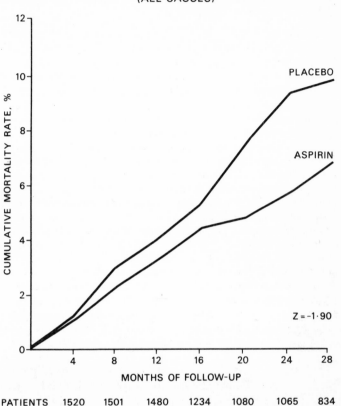

RESULTS OF THE CDPA STUDY

LIFE TABLE CUMULATIVE RATES FOR DEATH
(ALL CAUSES)

| PATIENTS | 1520 | 1501 | 1480 | 1234 | 1080 | 1065 | 834 |

placebo. This trial involves patients in Britain as well as America, and in Germany and Austria a similar trial of aspirin has been taking place since 1970, involving 946 patients.

Studies have also been made of the role of aspirin in preventing venous and arterio-vascular diseases. These led Dr D. Loew of Bayer AG, the German pharmaceutical company, to announce at the 1977 Aspirin Symposium: 'Under ASA (acetylsalicylic acid) treatment, fewer secondary myocardial infarctions and sudden deaths were observed than under placebo. . . . Our results, to date, also justify the prophylactic use of ASA in venous and arterial disease.'

The final place of aspirin in the battle against heart and artery disease has yet to emerge: but the indications look highly promising. There exists, also, another exciting prospect for aspirin in the future. One in three women who die from breast cancer – in other words, about ten women a day in Britain – die because the malignant growth has spread to their bones. At the British Medical Association's Scientific Meeting in Hull in 1974, Dr T. J. Powles of the Royal Marsden Hospital reported that test-tube studies with cells had indicated that aspirin might prevent this secondary growth and that he had started a trial on patients to test this theory.

There was *in vitro* evidence, he said, that 60 per cent of breast cancers tested produced and released osteolytic substances. Patients from whom these tumours were released had been followed up. Bone metastases and/or hypercalcaemia had developed only in those with 'active' tumours. The osteolytic and hypercalcaemic activity in some of the 'active' tumours was comparable with that of parathyroid tissue.

From their studies it appeared that prostaglandin synthesis and release by the tumours was the likely mechanism involved in tumour-induced osteolysis. Since aspirin was thought to inhibit prostaglandin synthesis, this was tested and found to have a profound effect on osteolytic activity of the tumour both *in vitro* and *in vivo* in animals. It also prevented hypercalcaemia in the animals but not soft-tissue metastases, he added.

As the effect occurred even a week after tumour transplantation in the animals, this suggested that the drug did not influence tumour distribution but acted on tumours already established in the marrow. This was confirmed by histological examination, which showed that although tumour was present in the marrow, bone destruction was prevented.

'This is an entirely new concept as far as cancer therapy is concerned,' he said. 'We may be able to control this disease by preventing the tumour homing on to its favourite secondary site.'

RARER USES

Aspirin has been used as an adjunct to insulin in the treatment of diabetes, and – as a gargle – to relieve some of the more unpleasant symptoms of glandular fever; it has also been used in the treatment of cholera.

Recently, aspirin has been employed to relieve diarrhoea in cancer patients who have been treated with heavy doses of radiation. In 1973 (*The Lancet*, 19 May), A.T. Mennie and Vera Dalley reported how fifteen women aged 47–65 responded. When conventional therapy failed, it was abandoned and each patient was given 900 mg of soluble aspirin B.P. ('Solprin') by mouth, four times daily.

In four patients the diarrhoea cleared up completely within twenty-four hours of giving aspirin. In another eight patients the diarrhoea was improved, although in two it relapsed forty-eight hours after improvement was first noticed, despite continued treatment with aspirin. Colicky pain which had accompanied diarrhoea in three patients disappeared during aspirin therapy, and one patient who had had severe nausea experienced dramatic relief.

Our findings indicate that aspirin may be of value in the treatment of diarrhoea induced by radiation.

Recent animal experiments support this possibility. The giving of prostaglandins to dogs induces diarrhoea, and the administration of Escherichia coli endotoxin, which releases prostaglandins in dogs, also induces diarrhoea; this is inhibited by the intravenous administration of sodium acetylsalicylate. Further, since prostaglandin synthesis can be provoked by many different forms of stimulation, and because aspirin at low concentrations inhibits this synthesis, we suggest that prostaglandins are involved in radiation-induced diarrhoea.

More recently still, evidence has been acquired by the Medical Research Council's Brain Metabolism Unit at Edinburgh that aspirin may be useful in combating a particular form of blindness known as retinitis pigmentosa.

On 9 July 1973, *Medical News* reported:

Retinitis pigmentosa, which produces blindness in middle age, now appears to be due to the harmful activity of lysosomes – the so-called 'suicide cells' – which have also been implicated in some theories of rheumatism. Their task is to digest bacteria and other foreign invaders but, in some circumstances, the enzymes they contain can be released to play havoc with the body's own tissues.

The trouble in this form of blindness is the presence of too much of a good thing, Vitamin A. This is necessary for producing pigments used in seeing. When light falls on the pigment the Vitamin A is released, but if it is released in too large quantities then the lysosomes are broken down to release their enzymes, which bring about harmful changes in the retina.

The report continued:

Retinitis pigmentosa now causes about 7 per cent of blindness, but the proportion is growing as antibiotics and other

drugs control other diseases. It first shows itself in night blindness in the 'teens, and the only treatment has been the wearing
of dark glasses, which cut down the amount of light reaching
the eye.

'Anti-rheumatism drugs could now play an important role in
fighting this disease,' says Dr Bill Reading (Director of the Unit). 'If
one of my children had it I would see he was given a large dose of
aspirin.'

Another recently indicated use of aspirin is in the treatment of
Erythroedema, otherwise known as 'pink disease'. Erythroedema is
more common in children than adults (causing redness and painful
swelling of the soles of the feet, palms of the hands, ears and cheeks),
but there have been signs of an increasing incidence among adults in
the last few years.

Whatever the causes – 'environmental stress', possibly in the
form of air pollution by heavy metals such as lead, cadmium or
nickel, has been suggested as a major factor – the victims suffer
considerable pain in the periphery of their bodies.

At the 1977 Aspirin Symposium, Mr Hilton Harrop-Griffiths,
Consultant Surgeon to the Royal Gwent Hospital at Newport,
described laboratory studies of the mechanism of the disease made at
his hospital and concluded:

> Environmental stress acts at the cell and organelle membrane,
> and results in the release of vaso-active agents. The main agents
> involved are the prostaglandins which have been shown to
> reproduce the symptoms and signs in patients with Eryth-
> roedema. Aspirin, because of its inhibitory effect on the
> release of prostaglandins, will mitigate the effect of environ-
> mental stress and possibly help prevent organic disease.
> Further studies could help lay the bases for the understanding
> of the unfavourable morbidity/mortality experience in indus-
> trialized urban societies. Such studies could explain the need
> for aspirin and other drugs in such societies.

THE DRAWBACKS OF ASPIRIN

No effective drug can be taken without some risk, however small.
Aspirin carries risks for some people. It can cause skin rash, asthma
or – in very rare cases – collapse, in allergic people. But only about
one person in five hundred is allergic. Sensitivity to aspirin may arise
quite suddenly, but usually in the company of other allergic
reactions as well. Because it is a well-recognized phenomemon, all

preparations containing aspirin or acetylsalicylic acid are so marked on the label: it is thus possible for the allergic person to avoid them.

Aspirin can cause dyspepsia. This may take the form of discomfort in the stomach, heartburn, nausea or even actual vomiting. The cause may be real – owing to irritation of the stomach-lining, or even a central effect on the part of the brain controlling stomach secretion – or it may be imaginary. Experiments carried out on some people who complained of aspirin dyspepsia showed that it was cured when a different type of tablet was substituted, even though the substitute was aspirin also! Other dyspepsia can be avoided by using only a soluble form of aspirin, or by grinding the tablets up in food or drink.

Aspirin can cause stomach bleeding. Much has been written on this subject – and much propaganda has been made of it by those with a vested interest in discouraging sales of aspirin – but what are the facts? My research suggests they are these:

In about 70 per cent of normal people, aspirin causes a blood-loss from the stomach and small intestine: about a teaspoonful a day on average during the period in which the tablets are taken. The blood is passed out in excreta and is not noticed.

This bleeding is probably caused by a high and irritating concentration of aspirin inside the cells of the stomach-lining. One theory suggests that the drug speeds up the rate at which the lining-cells of the stomach are naturally cast off, and that this eventually produces bleeding. When this phenomenon was investigated, tests suggested that bleeding occurred – on average – when six tablets a day were taken for several days before the test. But bleeding *can* follow the taking of a single aspirin tablet.

It should, however, be remembered that, though even a very small blood-loss may sound important to the lay person, doctors know that in normal, healthy people taking no drugs at all a small amount of blood is lost every day from the stomach and intestine, being passed out with the motions. Aspirin simply exaggerates what is a normal phenomenon. Furthermore, the loss may be reduced or avoided by taking soluble or enteric-coated aspirin.

For most people, then, such blood-loss is harmless. But for others it can be more serious. If aspirin were to be taken every day, for weeks or months, by a person in whom the loss is *above* average, then anaemia might eventually develop. It has been estimated that 6 per cent of patients entering hospital with iron-deficiency anaemia were thought to have aspirin-taking as the main cause of their anaemia.

Some people react even more violently. On 2 June 1973, *The Pharmaceutical Journal* reported:

> It has been estimated that 7,000 people per year are treated in hospital for the vomiting of blood as a result of the taking of aspirin. Most of the patients get better quite quickly by blood transfusion, although that may use up many thousands of pints of blood per year. The late Professor Macgregor commented: 'No matter how safe the drug [aspirin] is, the more that is sold of it, the more people we can expect to find ill through taking it.'

The Journal went on to deplore the fact that aspirin could be freely bought from places other than a pharmacy. However, careful investigation has shown that aspirin is associated with no more than 12 to 50 per cent of all big bleeds from the stomach. (The fact that no one is sure of the exact percentage simply reflects the difficulties of proving a connection; indeed, some experts still deny there *is* a connection, and even more doubt that there is a cause-and-effect connection.)

There is no relation between these big bleeds and aspirin dyspepsia; and the people who experience a big bleed after aspirin may never bleed again, even though they may take the drug again. This, indeed, is why some extra factor, not just aspirin alone, probably has to be present before massive bleeding occurs.

Some recent work in Glasgow suggests that one extra factor tending to prolong bleeding may be a relative lack of Vitamin C in the body, which is known to be associated with an increased liability to bleed. Another suggestion is that the patient's psychological state 'loads the gun', and aspirin merely 'pulls the trigger'.

In his paper to the 'Aspirin Symposium' in 1975, Dr Gordon Fryers referred to the big-bleed phenomenon like this:

> We know that most of those who have no demonstrable cause for their bleeding haven't taken aspirin. What disease have they got? 'Disease X'? If we follow the above logic, then any effect aspirin may have would be expected to be the inhibition of the defence mechanism evoked by the body against 'Disease X'.
>
> Is it, for instance, possible that bleeders from 'Disease X' are more likely to be admitted to hospital if they block some of their defences with aspirin?
>
> That aspirin is itself a cause of overt haematemesis or melaena in well persons taking ordinary dosage is far from clear. The huge effort that has gone into trying to overcome the alleged risk of aspirin causing major bleeding, and which has led nowhere, is going to

remain unproductive until a cause-and-effect relationship has been established and a test derived from it.

How much work has been done to identify 'Disease X' and find its cause and treatment? I know of none. Surely this is the fruitful end to attack? The disease must exist, for roughly two-thirds of acute ulcer bleeders have not taken a provocative medicine, and roughly a quarter would have taken an analgesic by chance alone. The allegation, therefore, depends on the selection of the controls and whether the symptoms of 'Disease X' are the sort that lead people to take analgesics: if so, the cause-and-effect relationship would be inverted.

Dr Fryers added: 'Just as ambulances take most sick people to hospital, but cause little disease, one would expect more aspirin to be taken by sick than by well people. One would not then conclude that the illness was due to the aspirin.'

To date, the largest survey of the bleeding phenomenon has been the prospective study carried out by the Boston Collaborative Group and reported by Dr Macha Levy in the *New England Journal of Medicine* (30 May 1974). This showed that amongst 25,000 hospital admissions, there was no more evidence of bleeding among patients who had taken the recommended dose of acetylsalicylic acid (ASA) than amongst controls. The only evidence of a relationship was in heavy, regular users of the drug – people who had taken it on at least four days a week for twelve weeks or more. 14 such patients were found among 88 who had no other recognized cause for their bleeding, compared to the figure of 6 which might have been expected from a study of 15,000 controls.

Commenting on this at the Aspirin Symposium in 1977, Dr Fryers said:

This excess of 8 was the only significant finding in this study in which 243 admissions for gastro-intestinal bleeding were reviewed. However, that is not the whole story because 57 per cent of the control series, who were heavy regular users of aspirin, took their ASA for headaches, whereas only 36 per cent of the bleeders had taken their ASA for this symptom. Could this difference have been due to their taking ASA for the vague symptoms that may precede a haemorrhage? If so, the real cause of the association found would be the reverse of that postulated.

Apart from gastric side-effects, some 3,000 people a year are admitted to hospital in the UK with salicylate poisoning – from other salicylates as well as aspirin. About 200 deaths occur each year, 80 per cent of which are deliberate suicides and only 20 per cent accidental. Undoubtedly, this total could be reduced if salicylates were kept in secure places in the home, especially in childproof cabinets or drawers – indeed, the introduction of childproof packaging in the UK in 1975 apparently brought about an immediate reduction of 75 per cent in the numbers of hospital admissions of under-five year olds due to ASA ingestion (*Lancet* 1977, vol.ii). But more stringent precautions have been suggested from time to time, including restricting the sale of aspirin to prescription only, or restricting its sale to pharmacists.

Would either of these controls have much effect? Probably not.

As Professor Neil Kessel of the Department of Psychological Medicine at Manchester University pointed out in 1965, after a survey of self-poisoning carried out in Edinburgh (*British Medical Journal*, 4 December 1965, p. 1336): 'The majority of the poisons taken were obtained on prescription . . . certainly in the matter of methods, the physician leads, the layman follows.'

It is not, perhaps, generally realized that aspirin, in one form or another, is regularly prescribed by almost all doctors in Britain and in most other countries too. One estimate puts the yearly total of aspirin prescribed by Britain's 23,500 family doctors as about 1,000 million tablets. So not only would restricting the sale of aspirin to prescriptions seem unlikely to affect the problem significantly, it might actually lead to an *increase* in deaths from poisoning!

Professor Kessel added: 'Control of the sale of aspirins by chemists and others . . . is only a small part of the problem.'

At the 'Aspirin Symposium' ten years later, London GP Dr Wyndham Davies summed up the danger like this:

> Misuse can occur, and the public debate is whether this can be prevented by a new and harsh policy of regulations and restrictions or by better public awareness of the prevention of misuse. Aspirin is becoming less and less popular for suicides. It was always cheap and readily available; but this is a special form of misuse. Accidental misuse occurs by children. This may be due to parents' carelessness. But this problem of medicines left around is not unique to aspirin.
>
> Patients' misuse becomes less and less likely as open medicine gains ground. Patients have a right to know how to use good remedies in a safe manner. .
>
> Doctors' misuse is due to medical education taking for granted that simple things can be picked up whilst rarefied

procedures fill the student's (and academic's) time. A medicine of such unique value and of such universal use as aspirin requires much more attention in medical training. It requires a lecture on its own. It is a stand-by of all good medical practice. It is not just another analgesic; there is no substitute that has stood the test of time. Therefore, not to use it when indicated, and to use some inadequate substitute is a misuse that is now widely prevalent. Not to be thoroughly familiar with all its combinations for enhanced effects, or its dangers in particular patients or therapies, is the major medical misuse.

Perhaps the last word may be left with Dr H. W. Balme, Consultant Physician to St Bartholomew's Hospital, London:

'In praise of aspirin,' he wrote (*The Practitioner*, June 1967, p.769), 'certainly it has its dangers, and a satisfactory alternative to aspirin is eagerly awaited, but unfortunately there seem to be no drugs in medicine that are both safe and effective. With all its defects, aspirin remains the first choice of analgesic drugs.'

6

An Armoury of Weapons

The oldest known medical prescription in the world is a clay tablet of postcard size, pricked with spidery characters, which some Babylonian healer put out to bake in the sun 4,000 years ago and which, literally, became buried in the sands of time. When, forty centuries later, an archaeological expedition uncovered it and scholars translated the cuneiform writing, they revealed a dozen remedies, including this one, for the easing of pain:

> Purify and pulverize the skin of a water-snake. Pour water over it and over the amamashdubkaskal plant, the root of myrtle, pulverized alkali, barley, powdered fir resin, the skin of the kushippu bird; boil; let the mixture's water be poured off; wash the ailing organ with water; rub the tree oil on it; let shaki be added.

Kushippu birds and water-snakes have vanished from today's pharmacopoeias, fortunately. In their place have come highly purified substances, potent beyond the wildest dreams of alchemists, and synthetic compounds tailored to order by the skills of qualified chemists dedicated to the conquest of pain.

An armoury of weapons is now at the disposal of the physician: mild analgesics for controlling light pain, stronger substances for tackling deeper disorders, 'knock-out' formulations for producing near-instant oblivion – all have their place in the spectrum of medicines today.

Martindale's *Extra Pharmacopoeia* devotes 240 pages to remedies for pain and lists more than 1,000 preparations. They range from over-the-counter opiates like Dr Collis Browne's Chlorodyne (to which a neighbour of mine became addicted, and no wonder, considering the active ingredients: opium liquid extract 1.4%, codeine 0.21%, chloroform 14%, proof spirit 5.75%, capsicum extract

0.032%, peppermint oil 0.05%!) to the most powerful knock-out drop of all, etorphine hydrochloride or Immobilon.

Immobilon has a potency 10,000 times that of morphine. It can – and does – knock out elephants. Developed in the pharmaceutical laboratories of Reckitt and Colman, it was first tried out in Britain on a herd of impala in 1963 and then flown out to the Kruger National Park to help with an elephant census. It was loaded into darts and fired from an air-rifle.

A. M. Harthoorn, the veterinary surgeon, described its use in his book *The Flying Syringe* (Bles):

> We chose a large elephant for our first target . . . we gave it 3.5 milligrammes (about one ten-thousandth of an ounce). This made him walk around in huge circles of a mile in diameter, but did not make him stop. Another milligramme did the trick and he came to a halt on an open grassy plain with the team standing at a respectable distance. It soon became evident that we could approach and remove the two syringes. Measurements were taken and ear-tags placed. . . . Eventually, a dose of nalorphine restored mobility to our 12,000 lb friend, with his estimated 80 lb of ivory tusk each side, and he ambled off into the shade of the nearest thicket with just a touch of a defiant swing of his head.

Happily, we humans are made of less stern stuff. Milder preparations suffice for us. For more than 150 years, from the moment the alkaloid was first isolated from opium to the middle of the 1960s, by far the most potent treatment for pain in man was an injection of morphine.

Morphine is present in opium in quantities up to 14 per cent by weight. It can, with skill, be extracted directly from the poppy plant; the procedure is known as 'taking poppy straw'. More usually, it is extracted from raw opium by the use of materials which include hydrated lime (calcium hydroxide), water, ammonium chloride, a source of heat and a filtering apparatus.

Although the alkaloid was first isolated by Sertürner in 1805, its chemical structure was not described until 1925 and was not finally confirmed until 1952. It was then totally synthesized. But the process involved twenty-seven separate steps and for this reason the main source of morphine is still the natural poppy.

It comes today either in the form of a very smooth powder, or as cakes. Morphine originating in Asia is commonly pressed into blocks and given brand-names such as '999' or 'OK'. Its colour can vary from near-white to yellow – or even light brown – and it has a slightly acid smell. Under the microscope, it appears as needle-like crystals which dissolve readily in water. For medical purposes, it is made available in the form of a salt – either as morphine sulphate, morphine hydrochloride or morphine tartrate. The white powder is usually made up into tablets or dissolved in water and sealed in ampoules.

The power of morphine to relieve pain has become legend. Weight for weight, an injection of morphine is about twenty times more potent than opium when eaten, and it provides the standard of pain-relief by which other drugs are measured.

Morphine not only raises the pain 'threshold' – the level at which pain is perceived – it also influences *attitude* to pain. It induces euphoria, which makes the sufferer more inclined to ignore the pain. It also sedates, often producing a somnolent state akin to daydreaming. But morphine can also bring on addiction; not only the mind but the body eventually becomes dependent on it. During the American Civil War, it was offered to the wounded with abandon. But so many soldiers became hooked on it that morphine addiction became known as 'Soldiers' Disease' or 'The Army Disease'.

In addition to the addiction problem, some people suffer such adverse reactions to morphine injections that they have to be taken off the drug immediately. For this reason, scientists began searching, late in the nineteenth century, for an analgesic as potent as morphine but without its addiction potential. For eighty years they synthesized literally hundreds of strongly analgesic drugs, many of them derivatives of morphine. But in every case thy ran into the same problem.

Heroin, for example, proved to be up to eight times more powerful than morphine and more rapid in its action. It was first made in 1898 in Germany by a process known as acetylation; in fact, its full chemical name is diacetylmorphine. Its basic ingredient – morphine – can be turned into heroin by a chemical process requiring only simple equipment: bowls and buckets, running water, a source of heat, alcohol, acetic anhydride, sodium carbonate, hydrochloric acid, animal black and a pump.

Once properly prepared, it is a white crystalline powder so fine that it disappears when rubbed into the skin. It is bitter to the taste and sometimes smells of vinegar. It was found to be less liable to cause nausea or vomiting than morphine, and to be particularly valuable in relieving the pain of 'dry' cough associated with cancer of the lung. Indeed, it is still a prime ingedient of the 'Brompton Cocktail', a variable mixture of heroin, morphine, cocaine and gin, devised at the Brompton Hospital and still administered for terminal cancer pain. But it was deleted from the *British Pharmacopoeia* in 1953 because of its addictive properties.

Next came pethidine, first synthesized in 1939. In tablet form, it was found to be about a tenth as potent as morphine but to have fewer side-effects. It enhanced the effect of other sedatives, and is still often used in combination with chlorpromazine or promethazine to make patients drowsy prior to surgery, as well as being administered as a local anaesthetic. But as with other substances related to morphine it proved to be highly addictive, and literally hundreds of doctors, dentists and nurses have fallen victim to its lures as a narcotic.

In the 1940s and '50s, scientific opinion began to harden into the belief that analgesic potency was inseparable from addiction, and directly proportional to it. As late as 1957, a medical author suggested that 'searching for a non-addictive pain-killer is a modern-day search for the philosophers' stone'.

This was soon proved to be wrong. A research worker in a Boston hospital tried blocking the unwanted properties of morphine by administering a known antagonist – nalorphine – simultaneously. It seemed to work. He then set up a study to compare morphine alone, the antagonist alone and a mixture of the two. To his surprise, the antagonist proved to be a potent analgesic in its own right. Unfortunately, it also produced vivid hallucinations and so had to be abandoned. Nevertheless, the fact that it had shown analgesic activity triggered a widespread search for other narcotic antagonists with a similar effect on pain. The most promising was pentazocine.

Pentazocine – based on the benzomorphan nucleus – was found to have an analgesic potency comparable with that of morphine, but none of the disadvantages of severe depression of respiration, constipation or urine retention. Clinical trials were carried out in which 7,000 patients received injections and a further 5,000 received tablets.

The Committee on Dependence-producing Drugs, of the World Health Organization, concluded that there was no need to control the drug as a narcotic, either nationally or internationally, and in the spring of 1967 – after eight years of painstaking research – the drug was made commercially available in Britain under the brand-name Fortral.

Since then, Fortral has proved very effective in relieving severe pain, such as that from a burn, fracture, cancer or an operation wound. Fortral tablets have proved useful in controlling moderate pain, and Fortral suppositories have saved many a night nurse from difficulty with elderly or awkward patients who cannot – or will not – take an oral analgesic or injection before going to sleep.

Fortral acts on the patient's total pain experience, which may help to explain why it sometimes produces hallucinations. Other 'magic bullets' in the modern pharmacist's armoury act in a more specific way. Some are tailored, for example, to the relief of muscular pain. They come in the form of creams, balms or gels which can be rubbed into the muscle – or on to rheumaticky joints – topically.

The more interesting, perhaps, is Transavin. Containing esters of nicotinic and salicylic acids, tubes of Transavin were taken up Annapurna in the backpacks of the British-Nepalese Army expedition which reached the summit of the 26,000-foot mountain in May 1970. In a letter afterwards, the expedition doctor reported that three of the British climbers had used it. 'One suffered badly strained back and chest muscles', he went on, 'following involvement in an avalanche. The second developed severe intercostal fibrositis, and the third had badly bruised himself after falling thirty feet and jamming in a crevasse. Transavin gave considerable relief to all three climbers.'

Relief from muscular pain or bruising can be obtained in a totally different way by the technique known as 'counter-irritation'. Various forms of counter-irritant have been in use since the time of Hippocrates: hot-water bottles, cold compresses, ice-packs, mustard plasters, and even actual blistering of the skin, have all had their vogue.

But in 1935, an American physician, H. Kraus, tried something more scientific by spraying the limbs of patients with ethyl chloride. Ethyl chloride came into widespread use in hospitals for the treatment of sprained ankles, 'wry-neck' and other strains, for colic, dysmenorrhoea, even migraine. But because it is an anaesthetic, toxic, inflammable and freezes the skin easily (sometimes producing blistering), it has never been possible to release it on general sale to the public for safety reasons.

In the late 1950s, however, organic fluorides were formulated to do the same job and these proved to be safer. A notable development was Skefron, which began to receive glowing reports in the medical press. Typical of these was one in the *Journal of the College of General Practitioners* (1963, vol. 6, no.180) from a Liverpool GP, Dr Eric Toke, which concluded: 'Skefron has, in a series of forty-one patients, shown itself to be a safe and effective form of self-medication which was of value in the treatment of myalgia ['fibrositis'], wry-neck, ligamentous sprains and muscle strains, met with in general practice.'

Since then, cold sprays of this type have found their way into hundreds of thousands of home medicine cabinets and into every trainer's bag on the football or rugby field.

Pains, like patients, come in all forms and sizes. Sometimes analgesics may not be the answer, or at least only a partial answer. In many conditions, relief is obtained by specific treatment with a variety of drugs which are not usually classified as 'analgesic'. Angina pectoris, for example, may be relieved by nitrates, migraine headaches by ergotamine, gout by colchicine or phenylbutazone, rheumatoid arthritis by cortico-steroids.

Sometimes combinations of drugs may be used. Many patients with chronic pain are agitated or anxious; others are depressed. For such people, to give analgesics alone would be insufficient. Phenothiazines such as chlorpromazine or thiorrdazine are useful in combating agitation, whilst trycylic compounds such as amitryptyline or imipramine can do much to combat depression. More will be said about mixtures later.

More than a quarter of all the money spent on medicines in Britain is spent by the public on remedies which can be obtained without a doctor's prescription; and 38 per cent of all such expenditure on 'proprietary' medicines goes on pain-killers, mostly for the relief of mild pain (Office of Health Economics Report, *Without Prescription*, 1968).

Of these, aspirin preparations have by far the largest share of the market. Some years before aspirin came into general use in medicine, chemists found that derivatives of phenol and aniline – compounds derived from the benzene fraction of coal tar – had an anti-pyretic action. Subsequently, they observed an analgesic effect as well. Although these compounds have never been used on the same scale as aspirin, they have nevertheless found a role in the treatment of mild or moderate pain.

The first of these compounds, acetanilide, was introduced into medicine by accident. In 1886, two physicians named Cahn and Hepp were investigating substances which might have an effect on parasites lodged in the intestines. One of the substances they tried was naphthalene. When their supplies ran out, they sent for more from the local drug-store, Kopps' Pharmacy in Strasbourg. Their order was made up by a young, newly-qualified pharmacist, but when they opened it they found that the substance did not behave like naphthalene at all. True, it seemed to diminish the colonies of internal parasites in their patients, but it also produced a marked drop in temperature – something which naphthalene had never done before. They questioned the pharmacist and discovered that he had mistakenly dispensed acetanilide. Acetanilide quickly became popular under the name 'antifebrin'.

Unfortunately, it was found to have a toxic effect on red blood-cells, producing a bluish hue in the skin and finger-nails (cyanosis), and had to be abandoned. However, at the same time as the relatively unknown Doctors Cahn and Hepp were experimenting in Strasbourg, there lived in the same town a physician of far greater eminence, Baron Joseph von Mering. Von Mering, whose researches subsequently led to the discovery of the role of the pancreas in diabetes, read the reports of the undesirable side-effects of acetanilide and decided to experiment himself. During his search for less toxic alternatives, he observed that acetanilide was converted by the body into para-aminophenol. He tested this compound and a number of its derivatives and it was not long before a new analgesic was formulated: phenacetin.

Phenacetin is made by treating para-aminophenol with acetic acid and then with alcohol acetophenetidin, and it has about the same analgesic potency as aspirin; it has, however, one major disadvantage: taken over a long period, it can severely damage the kidneys.

A friend of mine, William Kennett, a medical writer for many years on *The Times*, actually died as a result of taking daily doses of phenacetin over a period of fifteen years to alleviate the pain of rheumatism. His kidneys had been severely necrosed. Scores of other cases of kidney damage occurred until, finally, the Committee on the Safety of Medicines advised the Government to ban the drug from public sale, after it had been in widespread use for nearly ninety years.

On 1 September 1974, the Department of Health issued the following notice:

The Order prohibits from 1 September the sale or supply of medicinal products which are for human use and which consist of phenacetin or contain 0.1 per cent or more (weight in weight) of phenacetin, except where the sale or supply takes place in a registered pharmacy and is in accordance with a prescription given by a practitioner. The importation of such medicinal products is also prohibited by the Order.

Von Mering's original investigation of the action of acetanilide and phenacetin also led him to test another compound, N acetyl para-aminophenol, otherwise known as paracetamol. Paracetamol is actually the form in which phenacetin is excreted from the body, but von Mering dismissed it at the time as being too toxic.

Perhaps as a result of the high esteem in which his work was held, paracetamol remained on the reject-list for fifty years until two American researchers, B. B. Brodie and J. Axelrod, defined how it worked in the body and read a scientific paper about it at a New York symposium. Five years later, the drug reached the British market under the trade-name Panadol.

Panadol was the creation of Bayer Products Ltd (subsequently to become Winthrop Laboratories), whose German parent-company had originally patented aspirin, and it was indeed helpful to sales of the *new* product that at about the time it was coming on to the market, 'scare' stories about aspirin began to appear in British newspapers. Warnings about the dangers of aspirin when given to children, and about gastro-intestinal bleeding, were plucked from the pages of medical journals and given front-page prominence.

Panadol quickly gained in popularity in Britain. But in America (where Bayer still dominated the analgesic market with its own Aspirin), no such trend occurred. The aspirin 'scare' remained a largely British phenomenon and one wonders why.

As paracetamol, the drug was included in the *British Pharmacopoeia* in 1963 and went into widespread use for the treatment of many painful and febrile conditions, including headache, toothache, colds, influenza and muscular rheumatism. Because it did not have an irritant effect on the alimentary canal, it was – and still is – used in preference to aspirin in patients with a history of dyspepsia or gastric ulceration, and in those suffering from iron-deficiency anaemia as a result of occult blood-loss.

However, as with many efficacious drugs, it was not long before an undesirable side-effect began to be noted.

On 27 August 1966, three cases of severe liver damage after taking paracetamol were reported in the *British Medical Journal*. One, a woman of 30, had swallowed 50 tablets; the second, a man of 28, had consumed 150 tablets together with a gill of vodka; the third, a man of 54, had taken 70 tablets for low back-pain after downing a bottle of beer. Only the last case survived.

Commenting on the reports in a leading article, the *BMJ* said, '. . . there seems little doubt that the drug is hepatoxic,' and added: 'There are theoretical reasons for regarding paracetamol as a potential liver poison.'

Soon afterwards, Doctors Jean Thompson and L. F. Prescott warned that a dose of paracetamol as small as 20 tablets (10g) could cause liver damage, and 30 tablets (15g) might cause death. Nevertheless, the public went on buying paracetamol in large quantities. Sidney Locket, writing the clinical toxicology section of *The Practitioner* in July 1973, commented:

> The eclipse of phenacetin as an analgesic was followed by the phoenix-like rise of its metabolite *paracetamol*. Unfortunately, in acute poisoning paracetamol does not behave like aspirin. Vomiting, which usually occurs a few hours after the tablets have been taken, is seldom severe or accompanied by other symptoms, and the patient remains fully conscious. This initial absence of gross disturbance not infrequently leads to a false sense of security. There may, however, be anorexia, nausea and epigastric pain. Case histories of acute paracetamol poisoning include liver damage (in many instances), gastro-intestinal haemorrhage, cerebral oedema and renal tubular necrosis.

By December 1975, *The Lancet* (in a leading article, pp. 1189–91) was stating:

> The hepatoxicity of paracetamol remains a serious problem and liver damage has been observed after absorption of as little as 6.2g (12 tablets) – not much more than the recommended maximum daily dose. If paracetamol was discovered today, it would not be approved by the Committee on Safety of Medicines and it would certainly never be freely available without prescription.

The leading article went on:

> There have been suggestions that incorporation of Vitamin E or L-methionine into the tablets would solve the problem, but this is not really the answer. The hepatoxicity of paracetamol is abolished by minor structural changes which prevent its oxidation to the toxic metabolite, such as N-methylation or placing the hydroxyl group in the *ortho* rather than the *para* position, to give 2-hydroxyacetanilide instead of 4-hydroxyacetanilide.

'Surely', *The Lancet* added, 'the time has come to replace paracetamol with an effective analogue which cannot cause liver damage?' But a month later, Doctors Roy Goulding, G. N. Volans, Peter Crome and Brian Widdop of the New Cross Hospital Poisons Unit, and Dr Roger Williams of the Liver Unit at King's College Hospital, London, leaped back to the drug's defence.

A total of 775 inquiries about paracetamol had been received the previous year at the Poisons Unit, they said, but 'the impression conveyed by your editorial was, in our opinion, more denigratory towards paracetamol as a therapeutic agent than the evidence warranted'.

The doctors added: 'Admittedly, although gross abuse by the deliberate swallowing of large overdoses of paracetamol can be accompanied by hepatic necrosis and sometimes death, most abusers recover and the morbidity for paracetamol in the UK remains substantially below that for aspirin.'

The debate continues.

Paracetamol, like aspirin, is sometimes mixed with one or more other analgesics to obtain greater efficacy and smoother action. In such combinations, the normal dose of each drug is reduced, thus reducing the likelihood of side-effects without decreasing the analgesic power of the whole.

One such ingredient is codeine, a powerful analgesic in its own right. Codeine is morphine methyl ether, a derivative of opium. Like opium, it is addictive, although only mildly so. The usual oral dosages for the relief of moderate pain are 30 or 60 milligrammes, taken every three to six hours; excess brings on nausea, dizziness and vomiting without much apparent extra relief.

In a review of the pain-relieving properties of eleven popular analgesics published in *General Practitioner* in March 1975, Dr Edward Huskisson, of St Bartholomew's Hospital, London put a codeine-aspirin combination ('Codis') at the top of his list for effectiveness:

EFFECTIVE

placebo (red the best colour!)

A LITTLE MORE EFFECTIVE

dextropropoxyphene	Doloxene	65mg
codeine	—	65mg
dihydrocodeine	DF 118	60mg
paracetamol	Panadol	1g
pentazocine	Fortral	50mg
mefenamic acid	Ponstan	25mg

MORE EFFECTIVE STILL

aspirin	Solprin	600mg
paracetamol		325mg
dextropropoxyphene	Distalgesic	32.5mg × 2

pentazocine		15 mg
paracetamol	Fortalgesic	500mg × 2
aspirin		500mg
dextropropoxyphene	Napsalgesic	50mg × 2
aspirin		500mg
codeine	Codis	8mg × 2

A selection of simple analgesics in ascending order of effectiveness. The approved name, trade-name and usual dose are shown above.

He also commented: 'Aspirin remains the king of simple analgesics. . . . Combinations of aspirin and either codeine or dextropropoxyphene may be slightly more effective than aspirin alone, but since toxicity is the usual reason for avoiding aspirin, there is little advantage in aspirin-containing combinations.'

Sometimes a barbiturate such as phenobarbitone may be added to the analgesic, which has the effect of allaying the patient's fears or anxieties; or a stimulant such as caffeine may be mixed in, to cheer the patient up.

Such additives have no effect on the pain itself and only a mild effect on the patient's 'pain threshold', the level at which pain is perceived. A fast-acting barbiturate such as hexobarbitone, for example, raises the 'pain threshold' by only 20 per cent or so; loud music played through earphones would probably be equally effective. But mixed with an analgesic such as aspirin, it can alleviate pain in apprehensive or sensitive patients by modifying their *reaction* to the pain. The two drugs together influence the total pain experience: the analgesic decreases perception of the pain, the barbiturate calms down the response to it.

On 22 October 1977, Merck, Sharp and Dohme, the US-owned international pharmaceutical company, broke the news to a conference of 3,000 British doctors of an entirely new analgesic – diflunisal. It was hailed as 'the first advance in salicylate chemistry since 1889'.

Diflunisal is a salicylate derivative which differs from acetylsalicylic acid in two distinct chemical ways. Firstly, it has no acetyl group attached to its molecule: instead there is a phenol group attached, with two fluorine ions.

To achieve it, Dr T. Y. Shen and Dr John Hannah, working at Merck, Sharp and Dohme Research Laboratories in Rahwey, New Jersey, synthesized more than 500 compounds. Diflunisal proved non-narcotic and safe in animals.

Dr Ken Tempero, Director of Clinical Pharmacology at the MSD Laboratories, admitted to the conference that nobody, at that time, knew how the new drug worked: 'However, we are in good company in this respect, since nobody really knows how *any* of the non-steroidal, anti-inflammatory analgesics work.'

'It does share the characteristic', he went on, 'that it inhibits the pathway that is involved in the synthesis of prostaglandins – in the same way that aspirin and indomethecin do. Whether all of these compounds work only because they inhibit prostaglandins is very much an open scientific question.'

Dr Tempero continued:

> The compound's chemistry and metabolism, however, are markedly different from those of aspirin and acetylsalicylic acid – although it is a derivative of ASA, it is not metabolized to ASA. Its duration of action is also unusual – we have documented the fact that a single dose will last in excess of eight to twelve hours. We initially tested it for six or eight hours but found that its maximum effect persisted through and beyond eight hours – so we ran studies, hour by hour, out to twelve hours and it lasts for over twelve hours. It has no effect on blood coagulation parameters (probably because the acetyl moiety has been removed) and it is uricosuric in every dose that we anticipate using clinically. Although it is highly protein-bound, it has a different pharmacologic profile of drug interactions with oral anticoagulants than does, for example, ASA.
>
> These pharmacological differences seem to have produced a better clinical safety and tolerance record – according to our human studies. The amount of analgesia produced is definitely dose-related. When we studied single doses in such conditions as post-episiotomy pain or post-knee-surgery pain, we could very definitely tell the difference in the amount of analgesia produced by 125mg versus 250 or 300mg given orally. However, all three doses shared the characteristic that, when they achieved their maximum analgesia, analgesia persisted for the long duration of action – although a 500mg dose provided more relief than a 125mg dose.

Considerable discussion about diflunisal followed the report by the Merck, Sharp and Dohme scientists – discussion which was relayed to groups of doctors via the medium of closed-circuit TV, and transmitted to ITV regional studios by London Weekend Television.

In 1978, the drug was finally marketed under the trade-name 'Dolobid'.

7

'Just a Whiff'

The evening of 30 September 1846 was warm and balmy in southern Boston but even the murmurs from rocking-chairs on the verandas had ceased, for it was 8.45 p.m. Darkness had driven Bostonians indoors to their oil-lamps, books and crochet-hooks, and there was barely a carriage about. All the greater surprise, then, for the occupants of No. 20 Silver Street to hear the creak of boards on the porch, followed by a knock. The door was opened to reveal Mr Eben H. Frost, obviously suffering terribly with toothache.

'Doctor,' he pleaded, 'can't you give me something for this tooth? How about some of this mesmerizing I've been reading about?'

The frock-coated Doctor Hayden led Mr Frost into a room in which the principal object was a red-plush dental chair with a stained spittoon. He asked him to be seated. The two were quickly joined by Dr William Thomas Green Morton, an imposing figure with a bushy brown moustache and whiskers, a dentist of repute and owner of the premises. 'Mesmerism?' he thundered, when the patient repeated his request, 'I have something better than that. Hayden, bring the lamp!'

A third attendant joined the group as Morton took a container from a shelf and poured some fluid from it on to a folded pocket handkerchief. 'Here,' he told Eben Frost, 'hold this beneath your nostrils.'

Frost sniffed vigorously, but a glaze quickly came over his eyes. Within a minute his hand had dropped to his lap and his head had slumped forward. The dentist went to work rapidly, calling for Hayden and the other assistant, A. G. Penney, to keep their oil-lamps well forward and shining in the now open mouth. With a firm grip on his forceps, Morton tugged out a troublesome lower bicuspid, swabbed around the abscess below and then gently centred the patient's head, cradling it in his hands for a further half minute before he stirred.

'There,' he said to his assistants, 'it worked.'

Mr Frost was helped to an armchair after washing out his mouth. As he sat recovering, Dr Morton prepared a document for his signature. It read:

> This is to certify that I applied to Doctor Morton, at 9 o'clock this evening, suffering under the most violent tooth-ache; that Doctor Morton took out his pocket handkerchief, saturated it with a preparation of his, from which I breathed for about half a minute, and then was lost in sleep. In an instant I awoke, and saw my tooth lying on the floor. I did not experience the slightest pain whatever. I remained twenty minutes in his office afterwards, and felt no unpleasant effects from the operation.

Next day, the following story appeared in the *Boston Daily Journal*:

> Last evening, as we were informed by a gentleman who witnessed the operation, an ulcerated tooth was extracted from the mouth of an individual, without giving the slightest pain. He was put into a kind of sleep, by inhaling a preparation, the effects of which lasted for about three-quarters of a minute, just long enough to extract the tooth.

The 'preparation' was, in fact, rectified ether and although it was not the first occasion on which an anaesthetic had been tried out, the practice of anaesthesia can be said to date from that incident. As a result of the *Daily Journal*'s report, the news that tooth-pulling could be made painless spread rapidly, and patients flocked to the suburban surgery of Dr William Morton.

A week after the visit of Eben Frost, Dr Morton received an invitation from Dr John Collins Warren, a senior surgeon at Massachusetts General Hospital, to demonstrate his use of rectified ether on a surgical case at the hospital. The opportunity was too good to be missed, but Morton found himself in something of a dilemma. He had already begun to realize that the method by which the ether was applied was crucial to its success – one or two of his dental patients had vomited instead of losing consciousness – and he had already switched from a handkerchief to a glass funnel with a tube attached, through which vapour could be inhaled from an ether-soaked sponge.

Would this work on a severely ill patient?

Morton discussed the matter with Dr Augustus Gould, a Boston physician with whom he lodged, and Gould pointed out that the ether was likely to become diluted by the patient's own expired breath. It was decided that an approach should be made to an instrument-maker named N. B. Chamberlain to fashion a more efficient inhaler, and a circular flask with *two* orifices was designed. However, by the morning of the hospital demonstration, Chamberlain had still not completed the glasswork.

Dr Morton spent a frenzied hour persuading Eben Frost to accompany him to the hospital to testify, in case the inhaler was not ready, but in the end it was handed over and the two men arrived only fifteen minutes late.

It was late enough, however, for them to overhear a remark which Dr Warren was making to his assembled colleagues in the operating theatre: 'As Dr Morton has not arrived,' he was saying, 'I presume he is otherwise engaged. . . .'

As the two men burst in, there was a guffaw from the medical students banked in semi-circular tiers of seats around the red-plush operating chair, into which a thin, pale-faced man had been strapped.

'I apologize,' Morton gasped, 'would you allow me a moment to assemble my apparatus?' The surgeon nodded. Morton went into a side room, stuffed a sponge into the glass globe, poured ether down one orifice and pressed home a cork with a notch in it. He reappeared. 'Well, sir,' said Warren, 'your patient is ready.'

The patient's name was Gilbert Abbot. He was a printer aged twenty, and had a vascular tumour on his jaw. He looked at the flamboyant Morton, with his upswept moustaches and fancy waistcoat, and closed his eyes in resignation. 'No,' said Morton, 'I want you to look over there. There is a man who has breathed this penetration and can testify to its success.'

He indicated Eben Frost, seated on the front bench, who nodded. 'Now, are you afraid?'

'No,' replied the patient, adding with some spirit, 'I feel confident and will do precisely as you tell me.' He took the tube Morton gave him and placed it in his mouth, breathing in and out evenly. His face flushed. His arms and legs began to twitch. Morton kept the tube pressed between his lips for about four minutes until his whole body slackened. Then he turned to Dr Warren and bowed. 'Sir,' he said, '*your* patient is ready.'

The surgeon worked swiftly. Insulating the veins, he neatly excised the tumour. Only the patient's legs stirred slightly. He sewed up the wound and washed the blood off his face; still not even a moan from the operating chair. A full six or seven more minutes elapsed before the white-faced Abbot began to come round from the effects of the ether. 'Did you feel any pain?' asked Morton. 'No, sir,' answered the patient, 'only some blunt thing scratching my cheek.'

John Collins Warren turned to his colleagues and students. Recalling the howls of derision and cries of 'humbug' which had followed an attempted demonstration of anaesthesia in his presence some twenty-four years previously, he picked his words carefully. 'Gentlemen,' he said, 'this is no humbug.'

Later, he wrote:

> A new era has opened on the operating surgeon. His visitations on the most delicate parts are performed not only without the agonizing screams he has been accustomed to hear, but sometimes in a state of perfect insensibility and, occasionally, even with an expression of pleasure on the part of the patient.
>
> Who could have imagined that drawing a knife over the delicate skin of the face might produce a sensation of unmixed delight? That the turning and twisting of instruments in the most sensitive bladder might be accompanied by a delightful dream? . . .
>
> And with what fresh vigour does the living surgeon, who is ready to resign his scalpel, grasp it and wish again to go through his career under the new auspices. As philanthropists, we may well rejoice that we have had an agency, however slight, in conferring on poor, suffering humanity so precious a gift. . . .
>
> The student who from distant lands or in distant ages may visit this spot will view it with increased interest, as he remembers that here was first demonstrated one of the most glorious truths of science.

Fulsome praise indeed! Unfortunately, it seems to have turned Morton's head. He immediately patented his apparatus and went on to litigate against anybody who appeared to infringe his rights. He developed a persecution mania. Finally, on 15 July 1868, he became so incensed over a newspaper article which attributed the first practical use of anaesthesia to another man, that he drove his buggy to Central Park, New York, plunged his head into the lake there, hurdled a fence – and dropped unconscious to the ground.

He died a few hours later in St Luke's Hospital, New York, at the age of forty-nine.

★

The 'other man' to whom the New York newspaper columnist had ascribed the first use of anaesthesia was Charles Thomas Jackson.

Jackson was a bizarre character: physician, chemist, mineralogist, geologist, inventor and drunkard, all in one. At the time of Morton's demonstration in the surgical theatre at Massachusetts General Hospital he was teaching chemistry in Boston. The two men met fairly frequently and there seems little doubt that Jackson advised Morton on the characteristics of different kinds of ether and how to prepare them. He recommended rectified ether – a product sold by a Boston pharmacist named Burnett – and Morton took this advice. 'But my obligation', Morton declared later, 'hath this extent and no more.'

Nevertheless, Morton's success and reputation drove Jackson to claim that it was he – not the dentist – who discovered the effect of ether and was the first to think of it for surgery, and on 21 December 1846 he wròte two letters to a scientist friend in Paris announcing this fact and requesting that they be read out at a meeting of the French Academy of Sciences. He also sent a paper to the American Academy of Arts and Sciences.

'In the winter of 1841–42,' Jackson claimed,

> . . . I was employed in giving a few lectures before the Mechanics Charitable Association in Boston, and in my last lecture, which I think was in the month of February, I had occasion to show a number of experiments in the theory of volcanic eruptions, and for these experiments I prepared a large quantity of chlorine gas, collecting it in gallon jars over boiling water.
>
> Just as one of these large glass jars was filled with pure chlorine, it overturned and broke and in my endeavours to save the vessel I accidentally got my lungs full of chlorine gas, which nearly suffocated me, so that my life was in imminent danger.
>
> I immediately had ether and ammonia brought and alternately inhaled them with great relief. . . . I determined, therefore, to make a more thorough trial of ether vapour. . . . I continued the inhalation of the ether vapour and soon fell into a dreamy state, and then became unconscious of all surrounding things. . . .

Jackson added: 'Reflecting on these phenomena, the idea flashed into my mind that I had made the discovery I had for so long been in quest of: a means of rendering the nerves of sensation temporarily insensible, so as to admit the performance of a surgical operation on an individual without his suffering pain therefrom.'

One might be more inclined to believe Jackson's claims had they not been made so long after the event, and had not the chemist previously exhibited signs of megalomania. In May 1839, he had claimed the invention of the electro-magnetic telegraph from S. F. B. Morse, saying that Morse had taken the idea from him during a shipboard conversation in 1832 when the two had sailed together from France aboard the packet-steamer *Sully*.

Jackson went to considerable lengths to obtain publicity for both these claims and, in the case of Morton, even had the matter raised in Congress. Before he died, he wrote a 'Manual of Etherization' and one interesting section in it concerns the use of ether to treat insanity.

He describes an experiment at the McLean Asylum in Massachusetts in which a deranged patient was given a mixture of ether and chloroform which 'cast him into a profound snoring sleep. He was kept in a deep sleep for many hours,' Jackson goes on. 'When he awoke, he was quite calm and rational and continued so for months afterwards, and was finally discharged – relieved if not cured. We have heard nothing from him since.'

Ironically, nothing was heard from Jackson himself for the last seven years of his life, for these were spent in that very same asylum – as a patient. He died there on 28 August 1880, aged seventy-five.

Ever since the soporific sponges of the Ancient Greeks, physicians and alchemists had sought a magical vapour with the power to lessen or remove sensibility to pain. But the effort took a quantum leap forward one spring day in 1799, when a young scientist named Humphry Davy deliberately inhaled nitrous oxide – and lived.

Nitrous oxide had been discovered some twenty-five years previously by Joseph Priestley, the Presbyterian minister and Yorkshire chemist who had also discovered oxygen, but it had been branded as a 'destroyer of life' by the renowned American scientist of the time, Samual Latham Mitchill. Mitchill, on little more evidence than a hunch, had advanced the theory that nitrous oxide was the gas of the devil, attacking living organisms, causing cancer, leprosy and scurvy, and bringing on fevers. He had sent his theory – written as verse – across the Atlantic to the English physician Thomas Beddoes for comment. Beddoes, a year previously, had founded The Pneumatic Institution – a centre at Clifton, near Bristol, for the treatment of disease by inhalation. He had appointed Davy its first superintendent.

Davy had invented a 'gas machine' for condensing gases and it was from this, on 17 April 1799, that he took a whiff of nitrous phosoxyd which, as he reported in the *Physical Journal* later, 'is respirable when completely freed from nitrous gas'. He then tried it on a cat. The cat sank quietly to the bottom of a large test-jar, then got up again after about five minutes.

He tried it on guinea-pigs, goldfinches, mice, rabbits, hens and dogs. They all survived. Then he tried it on men – doctors and scientists including Peter Roget, who came through sufficiently unscathed to go on to compile his famous *Thesaurus*.

'From the strong inclination of those who have been pleasantly affected by the gas to inhale it again,' observed Davy, 'it is evident that the pleasure produced is not lost but that it mingles with the mass of feelings and becomes intellectual pleasure and hope.'

Of his own tests, he said: 'I have often felt very great pleasure when breathing it alone, in darkness and in silence, occupied only by ideal existence. . . . Whenever I have breathed the gas after excitement from moral or physical causes, the delight has been both intense and sublime.'

A few weeks later, he took a moonlight stroll along the banks of the Avon, returned to his laboratory and prepared six quarts of nitrous oxide. He inhaled deeply.

'The thrilling was very rapidly produced,' he reported afterwards.

The pleasurable sensation was at first local, and perceived in the lips and about the cheeks. It gradually, however, diffused itself over the whole body and, in the middle of the experiment, was so intense and pure as to absorb existence. At this moment, and not before, I lost consciousness. It was, however, quickly restored and I endeavoured to make a bystander acquainted with the pleasure I experienced by laughing and stamping.

'Laughing gas', as nitrous oxide was subsequently nicknamed, did not immediately excite interest amongst the medical profession. Indeed, Davy himself looked back later on his experiments with it with some disdain, calling his work on it 'misemployed'. But his book *Researches, Chemical and Philosophical; Chiefly Concerning Nitrous Oxide, or Dephlogisticated Nitrous Air, and its Respiration* – written in 1800 – contains a portentous passage: 'As nitrous oxide in its extensive operation appears capable of destroying physical pain, it may probably be used with advantage during surgical operations in which no great effusion of blood takes place.'

Yet forty-four years were to elapse before it was. . . .

The scene is an outhouse adjoining a doctor's surgery in the village of Ludlow, Shropshire. A man in skin-tight grey trousers, short black jacket and flowered, silk waistcoat is bent over a wooden table near the window. There is straw on the floor, a bowl of water and a cloth, a kettle on a stove, and bottles of varying sizes, shapes and colours on two small shelves.

The man bends down and lifts a puppy from the straw. It is one month old. Gently, he places it on a circular wooden plate and then covers it with a large glass dome. He waits. From time to time, he presses down on the glass to steady it because the puppy is wriggling.

After seventeen minutes all movement ceases under the dome. The man takes a sharp knife, lifts the cover and cuts off one of the puppy's ears. The puppy does not moan or twitch. There is no bleeding. The man removes the glass cover. Minutes later, however, the puppy stirs again and within a further thirty minutes is back on the floor, drinking water from the bowl and tousling the straw. The man makes notes in a book.

His name is Henry Hickman. A small brass plate on a nearby door reveals the true nature of his character: 'At home every Tuesday from 10 o'clock until 4, for the purpose of giving advice *gratis* to the poor and labouring people.' The year is 1823 and the slim Dr Hickman is just twenty-three. The incident I have described is depicted in an oil painting now hanging in the Wellcome Museum of Medical History in London.

Henry Hickman quickly realized that it was not safe to deprive an animal of air in order to make it insensible: something had to be supplied in its place. He tried carbon dioxide, introducing it through a tube placed under the edge of the glass cover. He was the first to show that it was possible deliberately to bring on unconsciousness through the inhalation of gas. Under his simple anaesthetic, dogs, rabbits, a kitten and a mouse all survived the removal of legs, ears or tails without apparent pain.

By 1824, Hickman was aware that he was on the verge of a breakthrough of real importance to medicine; to be able to spare patients the pain of the surgeon's knife would be a boon to humanity indeed. But he also realized that as an unknown country doctor he had little chance of acquiring suitable human subjects on whom to try out his gassing technique. He had no laboratory. He had no witnesses of repute. He had not published details of his experiments in medical journals; and he was only a young man.

Hickman decided on a bold gamble. He would write to the Royal Society. If the Royal Society were to recognize the value of his work he would need no further testimony. Through his Shropshire practice he had struck up an acquaintance with Thomas Knight, whom Hickman believed to be 'one of the presidents' of the Royal Society.

Unfortunately, he was President of the Royal Horticultural Society, and merely a Fellow of the Royal Society, but he nonetheless had access to the then President – none other than Sir Humphry Davy. Hickman felt sure that through Knight he would be able to reach Davy, whose interest in gas inhalation was, of course, well known.

On 21 February 1824, Hickman sent a letter to Knight describing seven of his experiments on animals. It contained this passage:

> There is not an individual who does not shudder at the idea of an operation, however skilful the surgeon or urgent the case, knowing the great pain that the patient must endure, and I have frequently lamented, when performing my own duties as a surgeon, that something has not been thought of whereby the fears may be tranquillized and suffering relieved.

Hickman followed the letter with a pamphlet in the summer, which he had printed locally. It was entitled: *A letter on suspended animation, containing experiments showing that it may be safely employed during operations on animals, with the view of obtaining its probable utility in surgical operations on the human subject*. It was the first publication exclusively devoted to anaesthesia.

Hickman addressed it to 'T. A. Knight Esq., of Downton Castle, Herefordshire, one of the Presidents of the Royal Society'. But the Royal Society ignored it. Sir Humphry Davy never spared the young Shropshire physician any of his time. And eventually, after four frustrating years, Dr Hickman wrote to Charles x of France, offering to demonstrate his discoveries to him and to his 'Medical and Surgical Schools' in Paris.

Hickman took the letter personally to Paris and waited. The King passed the letter to one of his ministers, the minister passed it to the Academy of Medicine, the Academy appointed a committee – and there progress ground to a halt. A British doctor coming to Paris with the proposition that insensibility to pain can be induced by the inhalation of certain gases? Only Napoleon's surgeon-general,

Dominique-Jean Larrey, was of the opinion that the work deserved further attention, but he was outvoted.

Somehow, nobody bothered to communicate the verdict to Hickman, who eventually returned to England a broken man. He died two years later, aged just thirty. He was buried in Bromfield Church (where he had been baptized), his hopes for mankind with him. Nearly a century elapsed before his perspicacity was recognized, in the form of a paper published in the American *Journal of Pharmacology and Experimental Therapeutics* and entitled 'The Anaesthetic Value of Carbon Dioxide'. Two eminent anaesthetists had repeated Hickman's experiments and found that he was right.

Two years later, the Wellcome Foundation held a Hickman Centenary Exhibition in London. The same year, a memorial to him was unveiled in Bromfield Church. The plaque reads: 'This tablet is placed here at the initiative of the Section of Anaesthetics of the Royal Society of Medicine as a centenary tribute to the memory of the earliest-known pioneer of anaesthesia by inhalation. AD 1930.'

Distinction at last – but too late. Millions had gone on suffering, and others had acquired the fame, in the interval.

The word 'alchemy' is generally reckoned to stem from the Greek word *cheo*, meaning 'I pour' or 'I cast'. And, indeed, the first alchemists spent much of their time pouring and casting, attempting to change base metals, such as copper or lead, into silver or gold.

But even in the first century AD, when primitive alchemy was being practised by Greeks at the famous medical centre in Alexandria, alchemists were more than simple, misguided metallurgists or optimistic wizards. They strove constantly to understand *all* the chemical truths of life, including those of the human body. They sought a cure for *all* diseases, an elixir of life, and they sought it by chemical means. They learned to evaporate, to filtrate, to sublimate, to distil and to purify. They invented stills, furnaces, flasks and beakers. And they made notes on all that they did.

There were Greek alchemists, Arab alchemists, Roman alchemists and Chinese alchemists. But in the Middle Ages, the teachings and practices of all sources of·alchemy tended to find their way to Europe. Thus it is no surprise to find a Catalan named Raimon Lully (or Lull) experimenting, around 1300, with a mixture of oil of wine (alcohol) and spirits of vitriol (sulphuric acid), and producing a whitish substance which he called 'sweet vitriol'.

He did little with it. However, two centuries later, an incredible firebrand of a surgeon named Philipp Theophrastus Bombastus von

Hohenheim – otherwise known as Paracelsus – rediscovered it in his laboratory and immediately gave it to chickens. They became unconscious.

'The following should be noted here with regard to this sulphur,' wrote Paracelsus, 'that of all things extracted from vitriol it is most remarkable because it is stable. And besides, it has associated with it such a sweetness that it is taken even by chickens, and they fall asleep from it for a while but awaken later without harm.' Paracelsus added: 'In diseases which need to be treated with anodynes, it quiets all suffering without any harm and relieves all pain.'

Paracelsus's work was repeated and written up in detail in 1540 by one of his followers, Valerius Cordus – who described how he used it to treat whooping cough – but the manuscript gathered dust in the Nuremberg city archives for at least two centuries. Then, in 1730, another experimenter named F. G. Frobenius decided to call his sulphur derivative 'spiritus aethereus': ether.

Ether became quite widely used during the latter half of the eighteenth century – and more so in the nineteenth century – for a variety of conditions. The French novelist Guy de Maupassant inhaled it to relieve his migraine. Dr John Collins Warren, who performed the first official surgical operation with an anaesthetized patient in 1846, used it for the treatment of asthma. Others found it useful in the relief of localized pain when applied to the skin. Along with nitrous oxide, it became popular with professors of chemistry who wished to entertain (rather than instruct) their students by intoxicating them. And it became popular with students searching for 'kicks'.

Michael Faraday, a student of Humphry Davy's, followed in his master's footsteps by inhaling gases including ether, and in the *Quarterly Journal of Science and the Arts* in 1818 recorded that 'When the vapour of ether, mixed with common air, is inhaled it produces effects very similar to those occasioned by nitrous oxide. By the incautious breathing of ether vapour, a man was thrown into a lethargic condition, which, with a few interruptions, lasted for thirty hours.'

Ether parties took the place of drinking bouts amongst the student communities, especially in America, and even circus-acts and travelling showmen began to administer the gas for the entertainment of the public at a charge of twenty-five cents per spectator.

It was after one such 'frolic' – as the ether parties became known – that a 27-year-old doctor in Jefferson, Georgia, decided to try some on one of his fellow party-goers who had a cyst on the back of his neck. The doctor was Crawford Williamson Long and he had inhaled ether many times himself, noting not only its intoxicating power but also its ability to render limbs insensible. Many times he and his friends had fallen to the floor with a thud, recovering to discover bruises on their legs or arms which had been acquired without a vestige of pain.

Dr Long's companion at some of these 'frolics' had been a patient named James Venable. On 30 March 1842 – four years before Morton's demonstration of anaesthesia with ether in the Massachusetts Hospital – Venable agreed to allow the young surgeon to excise his cyst under the influence of the anaesthetic. The operation was a success, as Long indicates:

'The ether was given to Mr Venable on a towel,' he wrote later, 'and, when fully under the influence, I extirpated the tumour. It was encysted, and about a half-inch in diameter. The patient continued to inhale ether during the time of the operation and assured me, when it was over, that he did not suffer the slightest degree of pain from its performance.'

In his diary he wrote simply: 'James Venable, 1842. Ether and excising tumour. $2.00.'

Dr Long did not publish an account of that operation until several years later. Had he done so immediately, he would certainly have been accorded the place in history subsequently given to William Morton and John Warren. He explained the delay thus:

'I was anxious, before making my publication, to try etherization in a sufficient number of cases to fully satisfy my mind that anaesthesia was produced by the ether, and was not an effect of the imagination or owing to any peculiar insusceptibility to pain in the person experimented upon.'

On the outbreak of the American Civil War, Long joined the Confederate forces and took charge of a military hospital at Athens, Georgia. He was forced to flee before the Union troops in 1864, but everywhere he went he carried a bundle of papers in a jar: 'my proofs of the discovery of ether anaesthesia'.

He died on 16 June 1878 from a stroke. His last act before falling to the floor had been to deliver a baby, having fully anaesthetized the mother first. With ether, of course.

'Roll up! roll up! See the stupendous exhibition of the gas that makes you laugh. Watch the vapour stir every fibre of the body. . . . See six Red Indians float on air.'

It is early on a summer's evening in Cincinnati, Ohio. The year is 1834. A tall young man in a frock-coat is standing outside the famous

Penny Museum, exhorting passers-by to see his first stage demonstration of nitrous oxide.

'Better than drinking liquor,' he cries. 'It's thrilling. . . . Buy
your ticket now. . . . Roll up, roll up!'

Inside, every seat is taken as the curtain goes up. There is an air of
apprehension as six war-painted Indians appear on stage and perform a short war-dance. From a side area, the young man trundles a
handcart loaded with apparatus, tubes and bags. He fills six silk bags
with invisible gas and hands one to each Indian. To his consternation, instead of showing signs of exhilaration and breaking into
uncontrollable mirth, the Indians fall asleep. One by one they slump
to the floor without so much as a giggle.

'Now then, sir,' says the young impresario, turning desperately to
a burly blacksmith sitting in the front row of the audience. 'You try
some.' He tries to force the gas into the face of the spectator, who
promptly chases him about the stage.

The blacksmith blunders into the group of sleeping Indians, who
awake and stagger to their feet. The audience roars approval, convinced it is all part of a prearranged act. But the showman grabs the
handcart and retires to the museum office as quickly as possible,
leaving a colleague to disperse the audience.

Why had it failed, Sam Colt asked himself (for the showman was
none other than the inventor of the Colt revolver, trying to supplement his museum revenue with 'gas frolics')? What had gone
wrong? Clearly, he had given the Indians an overdose.

Colt, astute in most other respects, completely failed to realize the
implications of his accidental anaesthesia. He decided he had better
abandon the practice of administering laughing-gas to strangers,
even if it had brought him considerable rewards in the past when he
had trundled his apparatus around the streets.

But the practice was continued by others, and thus it was, ten
years later, that a thirty-year-old New Englander named Gardner
Quincy Cotton found himself collecting $535 from a public lecture
during which he demonstrated the effects of nitrous oxide on volunteers from his audience. Gardner Cotton was still a medical student,
and he gave the lecture to help pay his tuition fees. This is how he
describes the events of the night of 10 December 1844, events which
were of great significance in man's battle against pain:

> On the night of 10 December 1844 I gave an exhibition of
> laughing-gas in the city of Hartford, Connecticut. After a brief
> lecture on the properties and effects of the gas, I invited a dozen
> or fifteen gentlemen who would like to inhale it, to come upon

the stage. Among those who came forward was Dr Horace Wells, a dentist of Hartford, and a young man by the name of Cooley.

Cooley inhaled the gas, and while under its influence ran against some wooden settees on the stage and bruised his legs badly. On taking his seat next to Dr Wells, the latter said to him: 'You must have hurt yourself.' 'No.' Then he began to feel some pain, and was astonished to find his legs bloody: he said he felt no pain till the effects of the gas had passed off.

At the close of the exhibition, Dr Wells came to me and said, 'Why cannot a man have a tooth extracted under the gas and not feel it?'

I replied I did not know.

Dr Wells then said he believed it could be done and would try it on himself, if I would bring a bag of gas to his office. The next day – 11 December 1844 – I went to his office with a bag of gas.

At Wells's surgery, three men were waiting: the dentist himself (who was suffering from a troublesome wisdom-tooth), Dr John Mankey Riggs (a fellow dentist who subsequently gave his name to Riggs's Disease or alveolar pyorrhoea) and the shop assistant, Samuel Cooley, who had bruised his shins the night before.

Wells sat down in his own operating chair. Cotton produced a rubber bag, tube and wooden spigot. Opening the spigot, he instructed the dentist to breathe from the tube and he quickly 'went under'. His colleague, Dr Riggs, tugged at the offending molar, and wiggled it back and forth before finally holding it triumphantly in the air between his forceps. Wells did not stir. Ten minutes later, recovered and gazing at his bloody tooth, Wells exclaimed: 'It is the greatest discovery ever made. I did not feel it so much as the prick of a pin!'

The dentist moved fast. He quickly persuaded Cotton to teach him all he knew about nitrous oxide and ways to administer it. Apparatus to make the gas and deliver it to the patient in the surgery was constructed. Further tests were made over a period of a fortnight. Satisfied, Wells decided to go to Boston and seek out his old friend and student, William Morton. He told him the news. Both men then consulted Charles Jackson, the geologist and chemist, who had once previously given them an opinion on a solder which Wells had developed for dental plates. But Jackson scoffed at the idea. Surgery without pain – ridiculous!

Undeterred, the two dentists decided to use Morton's connections with the Massachusetts General Hospital to gain an audience with John Collins Warren, the surgeon. Eventually, Warren invited Wells to his lecture theatre. The invitation seems to have been a reluctant one: 'There is a gentleman here', he is reported to have said, 'who pretends he has got something which will destroy pain in a surgical operation. He wants to address you. If any of you would like to hear him, you may do so.'

Warren was a formidable figure and his students undoubtedly took their line from the tone of his voice. There were suppressed smiles as Dr Wells told his story, and giggles as a volunteer stepped forward with a bad tooth, willing to submit to 'painless extraction'.

Exactly what happened will never be known. Whether Wells was unnerved and tried to extract the tooth too soon, or whether he administered too little of the gas – or whether the young student decided to play to his sceptical audience by feigning – is something only that anonymous volunteer could have said for sure. The boy screamed – and went on screaming – in apparent agony. His fellow students jeered the dentist, who left the lecture room with howls of derision ringing in his ears. His friend, William Morton, subsequently to brave a similar scene two years later with the same surgeon but a different set of students, tried to console him, but to no avail.

Wells returned to Hartford.

His failure to convince medical men of the value of nitrous oxide in surgery did not deter him from using it in dentistry, and over the next twelve months no fewer than forty-five of his patients (including a bishop and his daughters) made sworn statements that he had extracted teeth from them painlessly after they had inhaled the gas.

Meanwhile, William Morton had gone his own way, experimenting with ether in preference to nitrous oxide. The Boston doctor had read in a book, *Materia Medica*, that the inhalation of a little ether was not dangerous and he tried some. Then he tried a larger dose on his wife's dog, Nig. Then he anaesthetized the goldfish. Finally, he tried it on two of his assistants, Thomas Spear and William Leavitt. When the two men inhaled it, they became wildly excited and physically violent. This puzzled Morton, and it was then that he turned to Charles T. Jackson, the chemist.

There was only one basic way to make ether: by distilling five parts of a 90 per cent proof alcohol with nine parts of sulphuric acid at a temperature between 127 and 140 degrees centigrade. The resultant distillate then had to be purified, and this could be done by adding lime and calcium chloride before distilling again. Unfortunately, not all ethers made in the mid-nineteenth century were scrupulously purged of their impurities. Jackson advised Morton that this was probably the fault of the ether he used on his assistants, and recommended one very pure sulphuric ether – 'rectified', before it was sold, by Burnell (a local pharmacist). Morton took his advice – and we know what happened.

Subsequently, Jackson – in addition to claiming the discovery for himself – demanded 10 per cent of all Morton's fees for the information he had given the dentist about the properties of pure ether. Morton went on to use the 'sweet vitriol' on three more surgical cases at the Massachusetts Hospital (including that of a Miss Alice Mohan, who had a leg amputated) and on literally thousands of dental patients. Gardner Cotton went on to establish his own dental association, with its sole objective the painless extraction of teeth under nitrous oxide (he carried out more than 25,000 administrations without a single fatality), and Wells took his apparatus to Paris. There he was greeted as something of a hero. But on his return to the United States, he found his old friends Morton and Jackson engaged in a public squabble. This, coupled with a narrow escape from asphyxia by a patient given nitrous oxide on the operating table, seems to have preyed on his mind.

He turned to experimenting with chloroform, which had been discovered by an American, a Frenchman and two German chemists in 1831. He inhaled large quantities during a week-long sniffing spree in New York, until eventually he became demented. Out of control, he grabbed a bottle of acid and rushed out on to the street one night, hurling the acid over a group of prostitutes gathered by a lamp-post. He was arrested, and put in prison to await sentence. On 24 January 1848, he anaesthetized himself with some chloroform which he had managed to smuggle into Tombs Prison, New York and slashed his femoral artery with a razor, just before 'going under' for the last time.

There is but one footnote to add to this extraordinary story of claim and counter-claim, personal vanity and blatant rivalry amongst the pioneers of anaesthesia; it is the origin of the word 'anaesthesia' itself.

Shortly after a description of Morton's demonstration at Massachusetts General Hospital was published in 1846, he received a letter from Oliver Wendell Holmes, renowned justice of the US Supreme Court. 'My dear sir,' wrote Holmes, 'Everybody wants to have a hand in the great discovery. All I want to do is to give you a hint or two as to names, or the name, to be applied to the state produced, and to the agent.' He went on: 'The state should, I think, be called *anaesthesia*. This signifies insensibility, more particularly . . . to objects of touch. The adjective will be *anaesthetic*.'

And so it has been ever since.

Early in December 1848, the wooden paddle-steamer *Acadia* braved the chill Atlantic rollers, and set out once more from New York for Liverpool on her regular run. Aboard, on that particular trip, was a significant letter, addressed to Dr Francis Boott of Gower Street, London.

Dr Boott was an old friend of a certain Professor Jacob Bigelow, professor of surgery at Harvard Medical School, who had been one of the audience present at Massachusetts General Hospital when William Morton gave his convincing demonstration of anaesthesia. Bigelow wrote in his letter:

> My dear Boott,
>
> I send you an account of a new anodyne process lately introduced here, which promises to be one of the important discoveries of the present age. It has rendered many patients insensible to pain during surgical operations, and other causes of suffering. Limbs and breasts have been amputated, arteries tied, tumours extirpated, and many hundreds of teeth extracted, without any consciousness of the least pain on the part of the patient.

Professor Bigelow went on to describe the administration of ether. His letter, dated 28 November 1846, arrived in England with the docking of the *Acadia* on 16 December. It was transferred to the Royal Mail and dispatched to London.

While Bigelow's letter travelled south, Dr William Fraser, the ship's surgeon, was travelling north to spend some shore-leave with his father in Dumfries. The method of his movement is not clear: it may have been the newly-completed railway between Lancaster and Carlisle with a 75-mile road journey to follow, or it may have been the Liverpool Steam Navigation Company's 450-ton steamship *Royal Victoria* which called at Annan Waterfoot, only sixteen miles from Dumfries. Suffice it to say that the young doctor seems to have arrived in his home-town on 17 December and, two days later, to have paid a casual visit to Dumfries Royal Infirmary.

Whilst Fraser was chatting to two surgeons, James McLaughlan and William Scott, a patient with a fractured leg was brought in. He had been knocked down on the Caledonian Railway. The fracture of the femur was a compound one and the surgeons, after examining it, decided to amputate. Dr Fraser, who had previously met William Morton in Boston and knew all about the demonstration of anaesthesia to the medical students, persuaded the surgeons to let him try ether on the amputee.

An apparatus was hastily rigged up and the patient was asked to inhale the gas. Subsequently, a house surgeon at the Infirmary, Dr Alexander Borthwick, gave this account of what happened:

'The man sank within two hours after the operation. The ether was tried in this case, but it was administered very improperly owing to the unwillingness of the patient to inhale it, and the feeble and unconscious state in which he was.'

Nevertheless, the trio at Dumfries may well be entitled to recognition as the first Europeans to perform surgery under anaesthesia. The confusion comes only from the fact that, that same Saturday morning, Professor Bigelow's letter to Dr Boott arrived in Gower Street by first post, and the doctor leaped into action. He showed the letter to a near-neighbour, a dentist named James Robinson, who happened to be due to see a patient that morning called Miss Lonsdale.

When Miss Lonsdale arrived, she was persuaded to succumb to an ether pad, and had her troublesome molar extracted without any feeling. She said afterwards that she recalled only 'a heavenly dream'.

Whether the London dentist or the Dumfries surgeons operated first has been a point of controversy ever since: it does not really matter. What matters is that Dr Boott also dispatched a note that same morning to Robert Liston, the eminent surgeon, who in turn burst in on another friend of his – Peter Squire, the chemist – who had a flourishing dispensary in Oxford Street.

'Read that!' he said, plonking the note on the counter.

'This is most interesting and important,' replied the pharmacist.

'Yes, and you must fix me up with something so that we can have it on Monday at the hospital. I have an amputation of the thigh to do, and we will try it then.'

In a trice, the impetuous Liston had turned on his heel and was gone. Peter Squire pondered a while on what had been said and, at that moment, his nephew came into the dispensary.

'Why not try it on me first?' volunteered William Squire.

The following morning – Sunday – the pair assembled a pumping device known as a Nooth's apparatus, and soaked a sponge in sulphuric ether. William lay down on a couch and took the mouthpiece between his teeth. At first, he coughed a little, but soon he became quiescent and then, finally, unconscious. When he awoke, he reported no ill-effects. 'I wish you to perform the administration tomorrow,' his uncle told him.

Next day, the two Squires arrived at University College Hospital and set up their apparatus in the operating theatre. The place was packed with observers, among them a young student named Joseph Lister, later to acquire a reputation which exceeded Liston's.

Liston himself entered in an apron. William Squire appealed for a volunteer to try the ether but, finding none, asked a hospital porter – a burly giant named Sheldrake – to lie down. Sheldrake inhaled some ether but quickly became obstreperous. Leaping from the operating table, he struck Squire in the chest, knocking him over, and then jumped among the watching medical students, arms flailing. Eventually, he was overpowered when he tripped over the top bench of the lecture theatre.

Liston brushed the disturbance aside. 'We are going to try a Yankee dodge today', he told the assembled company, 'for making men insensible.'

The patient, a London butler named Frederick Churchill, was brought in. Squire applied his anaesthetic. The butler fell still. Grasping an artery with his left hand and compressing it, the surgeon cut and then sawed the diseased thigh with his right. Ligatures were tied and the wound covered with a towel. Only then did Liston pause. That night, he penned this reply to Francis Boott:

> My Dear Sir,
>
> I tried the ether inhalation today in a case of amputation of the thigh, and in another requiring evulsion of both sides of the great toe-nail, one of the most painful operations in surgery, and with the most perfect and satisfactory results.
>
> It is a very great matter to be able, thus, to destroy sensibility to such an extent and without, apparently, any bad result. It is a fine thing for operating surgeons, and I thank you most sincerely for the early information you were so kind to give me of it.
>
> Yours faithfully,
>
> Robert Liston

That night the surgeon went out to dinner. So overwhelmed was he by the events of the day that he persuaded the entire dinner party to return to his hospital and watch him anaesthetize his assistant, William Cadge. From that moment, he never again performed major surgery without the use of ether. His forecast that 'in six months, no operation will be performed without this previous preparation' was proved correct as news of the technique spread across Europe and even into Russia. Unfortunately, Liston himself had little time to appreciate his own perspicacity: he died of an aortic aneurysm within a year.

Dr Samuel Guthrie Jr. had a do-it-yourself mentality. To launch himself into medical practice, he vaccinated his own cousin. When money became short, he turned his hand to anything for which he might have to pay tradesmen. He became, in turn, lumberjack, gardener, stone-mason, carpenter, coppersmith, tinker and black-smith. He invented a priming powder for muskets, known as the Percussion Pill, which needed only a blow from a hammer to set it off and dispensed with flint and tinderbox. He read voraciously. He also built his own chemical laboratory and installed therein a still.

In 1831, the middle-aged Dr Guthrie dispatched a very important letter from his home at Sackett's Harbour, New York State, to Dr Benjamin Silliman, editor of a chemistry reference book known as *Silliman's Elements of Chemistry*. It was entitled 'New methods of preparing a spiritous solution of Chloric Ether'. It described how chloric ether could be obtained by distilling three pounds of chloride of lime and two gallons of 'well-flavoured' alcohol in a 'clean, copper still', and advised that it should be quickly corked up in glass bottles 'when the product ceases to come highly sweet and aromatic'. Dr Guthrie went on:

> During the last six months, a great number of persons have drunk of the solution of chloric ether in my laboratory, not only very freely but frequently to the point of intoxication; and, so far as I have observed, it has appeared to be singularly grateful, both to the palate and the stomach, producing promptly a lively flow of animal spirits and consequent loquacity.

When the letter was published, Silliman added the comment that Guthrie's method of preparation was 'ingenious, economic and original' and that 'as chlorine possesses so many peculiar powers, it is not impossible that this combination may prove curative or restorative.'

Guthrie believed the had merely discovered a cheap way to make a substance known to pharmacy as 'Oil of Dutch Chemists'. In reality, he had discovered chloroform. Simultaneously, in France and in Germany, other chemists were discovering chloroform independently. Exactly who was first is not clear. Guthrie called his, 'sweet whiskey' and friends sought intoxication from it in the manner of the ether 'frolics'.

News of the potency of chloroform spread until in 1847 a bottle of it reached the house of the then professor of midwifery at Edinburgh, James Young Simpson. Simpson was what today might be called a 'fashionable' gynaecologist. Anything he may have lacked in ability as an obstetrician was made up for in the gift of the gab. His fluency of writing produced a torrent of medical publications – on hematocele, uterine cancer, pelvic cellulitis, hermaphroditism, acupressure – the subjects became too numerous for many of his contemporaries to keep pace with. His dinner parties became legend. It was at one of these, on the evening of 4 November 1847, that the company assembled (Simpson, his wife, her niece, a naval officer and two of Simpson's assistants) decided to try a little experiment.

Simpson had been using ether in his obstetrics practice for nearly ten months. But he had quickly observed its disadvantages: the persistent and rather disagreeable smell, the large quantity needed, and its tendency to irritate the lungs and cause coughing on first inhalation. So he had tried other substances: iodoform, benzine, nitrate of oxide of ethyl, acetone, chloride of hydrocarbon. One by one, he and his two assistants, Dr George Keith and Dr Matthews Duncan, had methodically unstoppered bottles obtained from a nearby pharmacy and tested the contents on themselves, taking care on each occasion to leave one of their number awake to act as observer.

On that night of 4 November, Simpson's house party decided to have a genteel 'frolic'. It was at that moment that the host himself remembered having been recommended a 'curious liquid', heavy and colourless, by a Liverpool chemist named David Waldie. A search was started for the bottle. It was finally found under a heap of waste paper. Tumblers were filled and the men present began inhaling chloroform. George Keith started to laugh. Matthews Duncan got to his feet and waltzed around the room. Simpson became tipsy, his speech slurred. The ladies giggled.

Suddenly, the men became confused and incoherent. Then, one after another, they crashed to the floor and began to snore. Simpson

was the first to come round. He awoke to find his wife's niece, Miss
Petrie, also inhaling chloroform and murmuring as she slumped to
the sofa: 'I'm an angel. Oh, I'm an angel.'

It did not take the gynaecologist long to realize that here was a
substance far more powerful than ether. He wrote a paper about it,
which he read to the Medico-Chirurgical Society of Edinburgh. He
began to use chloroform in midwifery, and his first patient – a
doctor's wife – gave birth to a daughter on 9 November 1847,
without pain and in just twenty-five minutes of labour. She
promptly christened the child Anaesthesia.

Over the next six days, Simpson delivered thirty babies painlessly. Then, on 15 November, he acted as anaesthetist while a friend,
Professor Miller, removed a bone from the arm of a young boy
doped with chloroform. Two further surgical operations in Edinburgh were watched by a huge assembly of doctors and students,
who listened eagerly as Simpson pointed out the advantages of the
'curious liquid': more pleasant to inhale, needing no special equipment other than a bottle and a handkerchief, easily portable and less
expensive than ether.

The news spread quickly. But as so often happens, the very
magnitude of chloroform's success brought stubborn opposition
from certain diehards. Postoperative mortality would increase, said
some: Simpson set to, and proved that it did not. There would be a
higher incidence of convulsions, bleeding, pneumonia or paralysis in
childbirth, said others: Simpson collected statistics to show that the
reverse was true. One by one, the medical objections were over-
ruled.

But there were also religious objections. Scotland was the strong-
hold of Calvinism, one tenet of which was that pain should be
looked on as atonement for sin. Indeed, in Edinburgh 250 years
previously, King James VI had ordered a woman to be burned in
public on Castle Hill because she had asked for something to deaden
the pain of childbirth. The Calvinists' favourite quotation, in their
campaign against the new anaesthetic, was taken from Genesis 3:16.
'Unto the woman he said: I will greatly multiply thy sorrow and thy
conception; in sorrow thou shalt bring forth children.' To which
Simpson promptly responded with a quotation from Genesis 2:21.
'And the Lord God caused a deep sleep to fall upon Adam, and he
slept: and he took one of his ribs and closed up the flesh instead
thereof.'

Round One to Simpson. God had been the first anaesthetist: Man
was merely following in his image. But the moral arguments over
chloroform went on for six full years (during which time an increas-

ing number of medical practitioners turned to using the anaesthetic),
until it was finally settled in April 1853. Queen Victoria by then had
appointed the fashionable and hardworking Scot a Physician-in-
Ordinary. The coming of spring found the Queen heavily pregnant.
Her other Physician-in-Ordinary, Sir James Clark, called on the
advice of a reputable London anaesthetist, John Snow, who was a
friend of Simpson's. Could the Queen safely be offered painless
childbirth? She could indeed. Victoria accepted.

Shortly afterwards Simpson received this letter from Sir James:

> The Queen had chloroform exhibited to her during her late
> confinement. . . . It was not at any time given so strongly as to
> render the Queen insensible, and an ounce of chloroform was
> scarcely consumed during the whole time. Her Majesty was
> greatly pleased with the effect, and she certainly never has had a
> better recovery.

The safe arrival of Prince Leopold – helped by fifteen drops of
chloroform on a royal handkerchief – was not quite the final accolade
for James Young Simpson. That came thirteen years later, when the
Queen bestowed a baronetcy on him. He chose, as his coat of arms,
the rod of Aesculapius. The motto over it read *Victo dolore*: 'Victory
over Pain'.

Chloroform is a colourless volatile liquid with a sweet smell and a
burning taste. Its vapour is about four times heavier than air, but it
becomes contaminated with poisonous phosgene and chlorine gas if
the exposure to air or light is too prolonged. For this reason, it is
usually sprinkled rapidly and then inhaled immediately from a mask.
It acts more quickly than ether. It also causes less nervous excitement
and less irritation to the lungs. But it does have side-effects.

Chief of these is the fact that it sensitizes the heart to adrenaline,
sometimes causing the heartbeat to become irregular or, occasionally, to stop. It also produces a fall in blood-pressure and depresses
breathing, which may result in acute oxygen starvation, especially
in patients who are undernourished or exhausted. Delayed
chloroform-poisoning may also occur, anything up to forty-eight
hours after inhalation, with symptoms of abdominal pain, vomiting
or – later – jaundice. Liver, kidneys and heart can all suffer fatty
degeneration, possibly with fatal results four or five days later.

Not a substance to be administered casually, then, chloroform;
and it was not long after Professor Simpson's initial demonstrations

that the first fatalities occurred. They were largely attributable to overdosage, and they occurred in America, Germany and France as well as in Britain, but they served to drive experimenters to try different methods of administration of the vapour, and different combinations of vapours.

Over the next fifty years, the science of anaesthesia progressed in small steps, with development of apparatus – rather than of basic chemicals – its main feature. The open sponge or handkerchief gradually gave way to mechanical inhalers, in which the ratio of anaesthetic to air could be more accurately controlled.

An Englishman, John Clover – who can claim the distinction of having anaesthetized Florence Nightingale, Louis Napoleon, Sir Robert Peel and the Prince of Wales (later Edward VII) – invented an apparatus which delivered a combination of anaesthetics in three stages. First, the patient started to breathe nitrous oxide; then ether; and finally a mixture of ether and air. Unfortunately, it suffered from two disadvantages: there was no provision for air to be mixed with the laughing-gas, and no way of removing exhaled carbon dioxide.

Other machines followed. Sir Frederick Hewitt, at the end of the nineteenth century, devised one which *did* allow the mixture of oxygen with nitrous oxide, although his formula proved only suitable for dentistry. C. K. Teter in America subsequently corrected this for surgery, but his machine had no means of calibrating the flow-rate for gases passing through it. In 1910, two new machines appeared which permitted partial re-breathing of the anaesthetic gases, and in 1914 a major improvement was made with a machine which not only measured the flow-rates but vaporized ether as well. A modification of this latter machine – invented by James Gwathmey and built by Richard Foregger – is still in use in some hospitals today.

But while many sought the perfect anaesthetic amongst gas mixtures, others were trying a different approach to the prevention of surgical or obstetric pain.

In 1906, a German obstetrician named Carl Gauss published a report at the University of Freiburg entitled *Geburten in Kuntsliche Dämmerschlaf*. *Dämmerschlaf* meant a state of 'clouded consciousness' or – as the Press subsequently dubbed it – 'twilight sleep'. 'Twilight sleep' was induced by injecting a combination of morphine and scopolamine, the plant derivative described in Chapter 3. It was originally tried as an anaesthetic by a German obstetrician named von Steinbüchel in 1903, but Gauss was the first to use it on a massive scale. After five hundred cases, he reported:

The *Dämmerschlaf* produced by scopolamine-morphine is able to limit the suffering of the woman in labour to the lowest minimum imaginable. This objective is attained without disagreeable secondary effects upon the subjective condition of the woman in labour, without substantial interference with the labour itself, without danger to the mother, without injury to the child.

An American magazine, *McClure's*, took up the story and was closely followed by several other women's magazines. Typical of the accounts was this mother's experience:

I didn't feel the injection of scopolamine, for they first used cocaine on the spot before using the hypodermic needle. Very soon after, I found myself growing drowsy, and in about half an hour I fell off to sleep just as naturally as I do on any night when going to bed. The next thing I knew I was awake and I heard the sympathetic voice of Dr Krönig saying all is well, and then I thought to myself 'I wonder how long before I shall begin to have the baby?' While I was still wondering, a nurse came in with a pillow and on the pillow was the baby!

The international Press printed extravagant claims for 'twilight sleep': 'a new era has dawned for woman and through her for the whole human race' was how one writer put it, but the medical profession was more cautious.

A morphine-scopolamine injection has the effect of depressing the thalamus gland, sensory cortex and respiratory centre of the patient, whilst stimulating the spinal cord, vagus and certain other nerves. It increases the tone of those muscles in the body which react involuntarily. It also has a remarkable effect on memory: a person under its influence may still feel pain but rarely remembers it afterwards. Unfortunately, it is an unstable combination of drugs. It has to be protected from light. It also affects different people to different degrees: the dose cannot be standardized, as Gauss discovered. He also recognizes that a patient put into a 'twilight sleep' needed constant observation and this put a strain on nursing staff. The injections could not be given at home.

Nevertheless, the optimistic reports carried by newspapers and magazines led to thousands of women demanding the injections for hospital confinements, and the technique was used extensively for a year or two in Britain, France and America, as well as on thousands of patients in Germany. However, many mothers became delirious and many babies were asphyxiated, before obstetricians settled for smaller doses than those recommended by Gauss.

A special conference called by the White House in Washington in 1933 concluded that 'while a certain degree of amnesia is obtained, no attempt is now made to secure complete amnesia as was done in the early days of "twilight sleep".'

Another promising path had petered out.

The idea of inducing anaesthesia by injecting a drug directly into a vein is as old as Sir Christopher Wren, for it was the architect of St Paul's Cathedral who tried this first.

Wren was a brilliant scientist as well as a surveyor and architect. He spent nearly twenty of his early years at Oxford, holding the Savilian professorship of astronomy for eight years; helping to perfect the barometer; discovering a method of computing eclipses; and among other things, evolving a hypothesis to explain the movement of comets. The 'other things' included a number of medical experiments. One, carried out in 1656 with the aid of his friend Robert Boyle (the chemist), involved giving opium to a dog.

Wren reasoned that if the narcotic were fed directly into the animal through a vein, instead of through the mouth, it might have a different – and perhaps more potent – effect. But how could it be introduced simply into a vein? The hypodermic syringe had not been invented then. With typical ingenuity, he attached a quill to a bladder with a piece of tubing, and pierced the dog's leg. It survived, although stupefied.

Wren did not pursue his observations; nor did Sigismund Elsholtz, nine years later, when he induced unconsciousness in an animal in Germany with a solution of an opiate. The whole subject lay dormant for two hundred years. Then, after the discovery of safe ways of transfusing blood from one person to another, interest in injection techniques revived, and in 1872 a Frenchman named Pierre-Cyprien Oré suggested intravenous injections of chloral hydrate as a way of inducing general anaesthesia.

Chloral hydrate, a hypnotic, proved to be relatively safe. But extreme care had to be taken over dosage, and there were lengthy 'hangover' effects. Alcohol was tried, injected directly into the bloodstream. So were ether and chloroform. But in each case the result was the same: brain and breathing were severely depressed and the effect lasted far too long. Sixty years elapsed before something better was found: hexobarbitone.

Hexobarbitone is a barbiturate. The first barbiturate – barbital –

had been synthesized in 1902, but it did not act quickly enough in the body to be useful for anaesthetic purposes. Hexobarbitone was different. It acted in seconds. Its action persisted sufficiently for a short operation to be performed or, if more time were needed, ether could be administered as a supplement. Its only real drawback was that it sometimes triggered muscular spasms; nevertheless, it was used extensively – especially in Europe – and it has since been estimated that something like 4,000,000 patients received hexobarbitone injections before a better anaesthetic came along.

The new one, in 1935, was pentothal, or thiopentone – since nicknamed 'the truth drug'. It acted quickly; it did not produce restlessness in the patient during the recovery period; and its speed of action and duration of operation could be controlled by the dose and the rate at which it was injected. In fact, it was possible to inject it so slowly that the patient never became unconscious. During this dream-like state, he or she could be questioned and made to open up old memories, hence the connotation 'truth drug'.

Pentothal was used during the Second World War, both as a general anaesthetic and – in lighter doses – as a treatment for battle neurosis; under its influence, soldiers could be made to uncover what was *really* worrying or distressing them. It is still in widespread use today, usually as a precursor for gas anaesthesia. An interesting feature is that the dose needed to produce unconsciousness generally decreases with age.

Professors W. D. M. Paton and James Payne, in their book *Pharmacological Principles and Practice* (Churchill Livingstone) give this description of thiopentone:

> A few seconds after the intravenous injection is begun, the patient may report a taste of onions; unconsciousness follows rapidly, but is often preceded by a sigh or yawn. . . . After the injection, the effect . . . usually lasts for up to twenty minutes. . . .
>
> Apart from laryngeal spasm, hypoxia, inhalation of vomit, and similar risks inherent in all general anaesthetics, there are a number which apply particularly to the use of thiopentone. Thiopentone should be used cautiously in patients suffering from blood or fluid loss, in patients with adreno-cortical insufficiency or Addison's disease, phaecochromocytoma, distrophia myotonica, or myasthenia gravis, since they are particularly liable to circulatory collapse. A history of porphyria, which is acutely exacerbated by barbiturates, is an absolute contra-indication to the use of thiopentone.

While pentothal was taking its rightful place among the milestones of anaesthesia, scientists continued to search for alternatives.

Eighty years earlier, some samples of Peruvian coca-plant had reached the Göttingen laboratory of the distinguished Austrian ·chemist, Friedrich Wöhler. Working in the laboratory at the time was a young student, Albert Niemann. Niemann was on the watch for a suitable research project for his thesis and, seeing the leaves, he decided to try an experiment.

He soaked the leaves in alcohol, treated the extract with milk of lime, then filtered it. He added acid to the filtrate and distilled off the alcohol. The result was a syrup. He separated the water and the resin in this, precipitated the residue with sodium carbonate and then shook up the deposit vigorously in a solution of ether. The ether evaporated, leaving behind a powder of glittering white crystals. Niemann tasted it. He found it 'benumbs the nerves of the tongue, depriving it of feeling and taste'. He called it cocaine.

The natives of Peru had regarded the coca-plant as sacred. It was used as an offering to the sun. When an Inca warrior was ennobled, the king gave him women and cocaine as the two most precious gifts. The queen of the Incas was also known as 'Mama Coca', and the Incas could perform amazing physical feats whilst sucking a mixture of coca leaves and ashes. The mixture tasted like tea. But it took the visit of an Austrian expedition to the mountains of Peru in 1860 – and the nose of a botanist named Scherzer – for the leaves to be brought to Europe and their secret exposed through the curiosity and imagination of young Niemann.

In 1862, another Austrian, by the name of Schroff, drew attention to the anaesthetic power of cocaine when used in man; and in 1868 a paper describing the numbing effect of cocaine on the leg of a frog suggested 'it might be used for a local anaesthetic'.

The drug caught the attention of Sigmund Freud, founder of psychoanalysis, who was interested in its action on the nervous system. And it was a meeting between Freud and a colleague – a young physiologist afflicted with a severe 'phantom limb' pain in the region of his amputated thumb – which accidentally triggered the sequence of events which led to cocaine going into world-wide use.

Freud suggested to his young colleague that he should stop taking opiates and try cocaine instead. He did, and the pain became controllable. Wishing to find out more about the mechanism of cocaine's pain-killing power, Freud invited a surgical friend, Carl Koller, to take some of the powder while he measured the effect on his muscles with a dynamometer. Koller was an eye surgeon and, for some time, he had been hunting for a local anaesthetic for the eye. Noting what happened to his own muscles under the influence of cocaine, he decided to investigate further.

He borrowed a gramme of the crystals from Freud and took them to the pathology laboratory. There, in turn, he applied drops of a freshly-prepared cocaine solution to the eyes of a frog, a rabbit, a guinea-pig and a dog. He scratched their eyes, pricked them with a pin, touched them with a cauterizing pencil and shocked them with a powerful electric current. Not one of the animals reacted. Koller knew he had found his answer.

He sent some cocaine in a vial to a friend in Trieste, an eye surgeon named Josef Brettaner, who was due to attend an ophthalmic congress on 15 September 1884 at Heidelberg. Brettaner responded by offering to perform an operation under cocaine at the congress. He did, and the patient declared to everyone present that he had felt no pain whatsoever, although remaining fully conscious.

The era of local anaesthesia was born.

Koller set up an industry to market cocaine. Peru began to export thousands of pounds of the dried leaves each year. Eye surgeons all over the world began using it. Others tried it in different ways: sniffing it at parties or injecting it into other parts of the body. Amongst the latter was an American research worker named William Halsted, from Johns Hopkins University, and he was able to demonstrate that almost any part of the body could be 'locally' anaesthetized by injecting cocaine (or, later, other drugs) around the nerves supplying the operative area. He tried the technique on more than a thousand patients before a terrible thing happened.

Halsted had conducted each of his 'localized' tests on himself first. Within eighteen months of the first injection, he began to realize that he could not do without cocaine: he was 'hooked'. Fortunately, his personality was sufficiently strong for him to be able to wean himself off the drug. Thousands of others were less fortunate.

The drug stimulates the cortex of the brain, increasing mental power and decreasing fatigue. It also produces euphoria and hallucinations, and hundreds of thousands of people in the nineteenth century took it for 'kicks'. But the addiction it can cause, the depression and fear which follow, and finally the convulsions, brought distress to many before its full dangers were recognized.

Amongst those who fell victim to the terrible effects of an overdose of cocaine was a French surgeon, August Bier. He had experimented with animals but felt unhappy about injecting cocaine into patients before he had tried it on himself. So in 1889 he instructed his assistant to give him a spinal injection. The solution was too strong. For three months, Bier lay paralysed and on several occasions came close to death. Something safer had to be found.

Substitutes began to appear at the start of the twentieth century.

The first was stovaine, discovered by a Frenchman. Then Alfred Einhorn synthesized procaine – subsequently manufactured under the trade name Novocaine – and the German surgeon, Heinrich Braun, introduced it into clinical use in 1905. Novocaine had one big advantage over cocaine: it was far less toxic. For that reason, it has survived; indeed, it is still in use today.

The modern anaesthetist has at his disposal a cornucopia of substances with which to dull or temporarily stun the senses: thiopentone, procaine, buthalitone, methohexitone, to name but a few which make the patient drowsy and co-operative; or chloroform, nitrous oxide, ether, trichloroethylene, cyclopropane, halothane, ethyl chloride or methoxyflurane for rendering him more deeply insensible. Individual anaesthetists prefer other agents.

The mechanism of their action is still not clearly understood.

Soon after ether and chloroform were introduced, several theories were put forward to explain how they produced anaesthesia. One suggested that they acted on the surface of the brain; another, that colloid was coagulated; a third, that they disturbed the oxygen consumption of the brain; a fourth, that they depressed the permeability of cells.

In *Pharmacological Principles and Practice*, Professors Paton and Payne prefer an explanation put forward independently, by Meyer in 1899 and Overton in 1901, called the lipoid-solubility theory. This points out that anaesthetic potency is correlated with fat solubility:

> If the concentration of anaesthetic required to produce some standard anaesthetic state is multiplied by its solubility in olive oil, it is found that the result varies between about 0.03 and 0.1 moles of anaesthetic per litre of fat, although the tensions of the anaesthetics used may vary from 30 atmospheres (for nitrogen) to 0.5% of an atmosphere for chloroform – a ratio of 6,000. . . . This is one of the most remarkable generalizations in pharmacology.

The two authors point out that the strength of the lipoid-solubility theory is that 'it generalizes to a remarkable degree the widely varying potencies of different anaesthetics, and that it explains why no particular chemical structure is required for anaesthesia. . . . Its main weakness is that it does not indicate the intimate mechanism of the anaesthesia.'

L. J. Mullins (in *Chemical Review* vol. 54, pp. 289–323) suggests that the 'intimate mechanism' may be one of physical blocking; that the key factor may be the molecular volume of the drug. A molecule is anaesthetic because it fits into – and blocks – channels in cell membranes through which the movement of ions takes place.

Linus Pauling (in *Science*, 1961, vol. 134, pp. 15–21) and S. L. Miller (in *Proceedings of the National Academy of Sciences*, 1961, vol. 47, pp. 1515–24) prefer the concept of clathrate formation. A clathrate is formed by 'molecular imprisonment': combined molecules are held together mechanically by virtue of their configuration. Thus, if a molecular of xenon lies within a chamber, a shell of twelve water molecules can form around it, the bond between the two being hydrogen. The xenon is imprisoned by the water. A similar thing seems to happen with chloroform, and perhaps other anaesthetics as well. This implies that a water 'coating' around the molecules of drug may increase the electrical impedance of nervous tissue and so reduce its activity, thus causing anaesthesia.

So much for the chemists' theories.

Neuro-physiological studies have suggested that the 'intimate mechanism' of anaesthesia may be a loss of efficiency in the transmitter at synapses in nerve-cells, and a decrease in sensitivity of the postsynaptic surface to it.

'The various approaches to the problem are not mutually exclusive,' point out Professors Paton and Payne. 'If one supposes that the uptake of anaesthetic by the lipoidal part of neuronal membranes leads to a reduction of synaptic activity and that, as a result, the tissue as a whole becomes less active, then the physico-chemical, electro-physiological and biochemical findings all fall into a single, coherent pattern.'

In their manual for physicians and nurses, *Obstetric Analgesia and Anaesthesia*, prepared in 1972, the World Federation of Societies of Anaesthiologists came to this conclusion about the mechanism of action of local anaesthetics:

> Local anaesthetics are salts, usually hydrochlorides, which combine a weak base with a strong acid. They liberate the base in the body where the slightly alkaline, extra-cellular fluids cause hydrolysis. The undissociated base penetrates fibrous tissues to reach the nerve membrane where it dissociates, producing anaesthesia. The dissociated base seems to prevent the ionic migration necessary for nerve-impulse conduction, probably by obstructing sodium ion inflow through the nerve membrane and preventing depolarization.

So much for *how* anaesthetics may work.

There are three desirable stages in anaesthesia, and one undesirable one. Stage One leads up to unconsciousness. The patient becomes less and less sensitive to pain, more and more forgetful; he can respond to orders because he can still hear, but as unconsciousness approaches so his reflexes disappear. Eventually, a standard test – touching the eyelashes – produces no response.

Stage Two is characterized by delirium. Anaesthetists like to speed through this stage as quickly as possible. If they fail, the patient's breathing becomes laboured, he sweats, his eyeballs move vigorously and he may actually writhe and struggle, perhaps vomit.

With Stage Three comes quieter, more regular breathing. It has a number of 'mini-stages' within it. For instance, at first the pulse-rate remains normal, and the pupil of the eye is still small and can react to light. At this level, all superficial and thoracic surgery may be carried out without pain to the patient. As the second 'mini-stage' is reached, the movement of the eyeballs ceases and muscle tone starts to weaken. In this state, surgery of the lower abdomen is possible. As the anaesthesia becomes deeper still, so the muscles go slack. Breathing becomes shallower and more rapid; the pupils of the eyes dilate; upper abdominal surgery becomes possible. A final 'mini-stage' can be reached where all chest movement ceases and the patient is breathing only with his diaphragm.

Stage Four is reached only inadvertently. Breathing stops completely; pulse-rate increases; blood-pressure rises steeply, and the blood turns blue. Finally the heart fails, due to asphyxia.

I always remember trying to recollect my own response to the stages of anaesthesia during a dental operation in 1953. I was about to take my Tripos finals at Cambridge and had developed acute toothache. The dentist diagnosed an abscess and told me to return to his surgery at 2.30 p.m., when he would have an anaesthetist present to administer a general anaesthetic. My last experience of a general anaesthetic had been fourteen years previously when I had broken my nose, but it had given me a clear memory of white horses charging at me faster and faster just before I 'went under'.

What, I wondered, could I remember this time? I decided to co-operate physically with the anaesthetist but to 'hold on' mentally for as long as possible. At 2.30 I breathed greedily from the face-mask until I heard the anaesthetist say, 'Open your eyes.' I did so. Through a haze I could see his face. 'Open your eyes,' he said again. 'They are open,' I wanted to tell him. Again, 'Open your eyes!'

His tone was sharp and sounded urgent, almost panicky. 'Oh God,' I thought under the influence of the nitrous oxide, 'something's gone wrong.' I decided to give him a chance to right things but, if he didn't do so quickly, to force myself back to full consciousness and wrench the mask off. Then I did not care any more. There was nothing I could do. I was helpless.

I died. In the aeons of time through which my imagination led me (actually it was about two minutes), I heard the entire coroner's inquest on my death, and witnessed the reactions of all my friends and relatives to it. Suddenly, I thought to myself: 'How is it that you have retained the same cognitive process throughout – from life, through death and now beyond? Why are you thinking in the same way as you were *then*?'

I concluded that I must have been God, without knowing it, all the time that I was alive. With that thought, I went to sleep. . . .

When I came round, I am told, I thanked the dentist three times in quick succession for resurrecting me and had to be treated for fifteen minutes for shock! What I had not known was that a standard method used to recognize the stages of anaesthesia was to observe the pupils of the eyes. All this anaesthetist had been trying to do was to test my reflexes. So much for the hallucinatory power of laughing-gas!

Nitrous oxide – first prepared by Joseph Priestley in 1772 from nitric oxide and damp iron filings but now made by heating ammonium nitrate – is still the most widely used anaesthetic in dentistry and was, for many years, in obstetrics. When a mixture of 80% nitrous oxide and 20% oxygen is used, few toxic effects are observed. But more potent anaesthetics have been developed.

Cyclopropane – first made in 1882 but not used clinically until 1934 – is more potent than nitrous oxide and also faster-acting. Made by heating trimethylene dibromide with zinc, and then compressed into orange-coloured cylinders, it can produce unconsciousness in fifteen to twenty breaths. It has been widely used in thoracic surgery and in cases of heart disease. Its great virtue is its non-irritancy. But many patients have experienced a phenomenon known as 'cyclopropane shock' during the postoperative period: clammy skin, pallor, low blood-pressure and a fast, jumpy pulse. It is also expensive.

Halothane – first tried clinically in 1956 and synthesized by direct bromination of 1, 1, 1-trifluoro: 2-chloroethane – does not irritate the respiratory tract either. There is little danger of the patient coughing while inhaling it. It can induce anaesthesia from scratch; but, more commonly, it is used after an injection of thiopentone to maintain unconsciousness. It has a smell not unlike chloroform, and has to be kept in amber-coloured bottles to prevent sunlight from decomposing it, but otherwise it is easy and pleasant for both patient and anaesthetist to use and has comparatively few side-effects.

Surveys of more than 30,000 patients in America who received halothane showed that it caused liver damage in only fractionally more cases than other general anaesthetics; a similar survey of 27,000 patients in Britain – reported by W.W. Mushin and colleagues in the

British Medical Journal (vol. 2, 1964, p. 329) – concluded that 'the incidence of hepatic complications after halothane administration is little different from that after non-halothane anaesthetics'. However, in a leading article in *The Lancet* in 1961, this warning was given:

Halothane relaxes the parturient uterus and the use of halothane in operative obstetrics is therefore dangerous. It also leads to significant depression of respiration in the foetus. Halothane is not always acceptable in neuro-surgery since it may increase cerebral blood-flow and increase intra-cranial tension, although the drug may have a place in the deliberate induction of hypotension in neuro-surgery.

Reports of bradycardia appeared. But it was found that this could be countered by an intravenous injection of 0.5 mg of atropine. Severe hypotension was found to be combatable by an intravenous injection of 5 to 10 mg of methoxamine hydrochloride; and respiratory depression, another occasional feature, was reversible by reducing the concentration of halothane and giving oxygen.

On the whole, halothane has emerged with a good record as an anaesthetic and has proved a boon to hundreds of thousands.

Ethyl chloride – discovered in the seventeenth century but not put into clinical use until the late nineteenth – is another agent which does not irritate the bronchi and is still in widespread use, especially for short operations or operations on children. Many a tooth, tonsil or set of adenoids has come out under ethyl chloride. It is a volatile, colourless liquid, obtained from the action of hydrochloric acid on alcohol, capable of inducing full surgical anaesthesia rapidly and smoothly. Children recover full consciousness within a few minutes of the end of an operation and muscle tone returns quickly; but its rapid action – plus the poisonous effects it can have on the heart and liver – make it harder to control than chloroform, and limit its use to short exposures.

Chloroform itself is now recognized as a hazardous anaesthetic because of its toxicity. It can damage the liver and kidneys and cause irregularities in the heartbeat and, 'for this reason, few medical students receive instruction in its use today; nevertheless, it is still in fairly widespread use among domiciliary midwives who manage to avoid most of its pitfalls by using a modern vaporizer known as 'the Chlorotec'.

Trichloroethylene, another favourite in midwifery, began its career as a solvent for grease in industry.

During the 1914–18 war, it was used by munitions manufacturers for de-greasing metal and also as a dry-cleaning agent. Sometimes an employee would go down with poisoning from its fumes and, when this happened, it was noticed that loss of sensation occurred in the worker's face. Research into its properties continued after the war, and in 1935, American anaesthetists introduced it into clinical medicine for minor surgery. It does, however, cause a rise in pressure in the brain, and the American Medical Association issued a critical report about it in 1936.

However, in 1941, the London anaesthetist, Dr Langton Hewer, published an account which revived interest in it on a grand scale. It is now used as an adjurant to nitrous oxide and oxygen mixtures – or as the sole agent in obstetrics – and since 1955, British midwives have been allowed to use it at will. A clinical trial conducted by the Medical Research Council has concluded that it is as safe as 'gas and air'. Unfortunately, a number of people have become addicted to it. Trichloroethylene has enjoyed greater popularity than a gas with a similar name but different composition: Ethylene.

Ethylene, too, became an anaesthetic by accident. Research workers were first put on to its trail by a chance observation by two botanists that carnations grown in certain greenhouses failed to open into blooms. They literally 'went to sleep'. They investigated and found that the greenhouses in question were being heated with a burner-gas containing a 4 per cent concentration of ethylene. Ten years later, another research worker looking into the lethal effects of ethylene on plants, tried some on a frog and found that it did not kill the animal but merely anaesthetized it.

Unfortunately, the gas does not produce deep anaesthesia and is only suitable, therefore, for light surgery. Furthermore, it is highly inflammable and cannot be used in the presence of machinery generating heat or a spark.

Experiments with ethylene in the 1930s, however, led Professor Chauncey Leake and Miss Mei-yu-Chen of the University of California to try crossing ethylene with ether. Ethylene, they reasoned, acted quickly but weakly; ether was slow but strong. A chemist friend, Professor Lauder Jones of Princeton University, was asked to prepare a liquid with these properties, and another anaesthetic was born: divinyl ether.

Divinyl ether has been widely used to render anaesthesia more pleasant. Divinyl oxide can be given at the start and then, when the patient slips into unconsciousness, ether can take over. It can be carried in the physician's bag and has performed valiant service in the lancing of boils or treatment of infected ears.

Methoxyflurane is the latest gas anaesthetic to be introduced on any scale. It was first tried clinically in 1960. It is a clear, colourless liquid with a fruity smell, and is non-explosive and non-inflammable. When used alone with oxygen, however, it is rather slow to act – anaesthesia can take twenty minutes – and for this reason, it is usually preceded by an intravenous injection of barbiturate and by nitrous oxide and oxygen. Anaesthesia is then usually maintained with a 75:25 mixture of methoxyflurane and nitrous oxide/oxygen. It is pleasant to take but slow to clear from the body. Reports in clinical journals on its use since 1960 contain phrases such as 'easy to handle', 'produced good muscle relaxation', 'did not interfere with cardiovascular function'. But all reports comment on the time it takes to act and the slow recovery of the patient.

So much for the gas anaesthetics.

As far as intravenous anaesthetics are concerned, their main advantage is their speed of action; their main disadvantage, the fact that injections may be painful or – if misplaced – hazardous.

Thiopentone sodium, a pale-yellow powder which dissolves in water, can bring about muscle relaxation in thirty seconds. It may also be dripped repeatedly into a vein for operations lasting longer than a few minutes. It is often used with curare, the Indian arrow poison, to bring about complete muscular relaxation during chest or abdominal surgery, and may be given in the form of rectal suppositories to anaesthetize the spine in small children.

Thialbarbitone is another short-acting barbiturate, only about half as potent as thiopentone, but producing less depression of the respiratory system in the patient.

Sodium thiamylal is about one-and-a-half times more potent than thiopentone and is often given as an adjunct to gas anaesthetics.

Buthalitone acts even more rapidly than the others, and permits even faster recovery. For this reason, it is often used with out-patients.

Methohexitone finally, is another with greater potency than thiopentone. But because it is less easily absorbed by the fatty tissues, larger doses are needed to maintain anaesthesia.

Each drug, each gas, has advantages and disadvantages. Each patient is different: a different size, a different weight, with a different metabolism. The anaesthetist, doctor or midwife has to make a judgement in each case on the best available evidence. But what a variety of agents is now at his or her disposal. Anaesthetics has indeed come a long way since Eben Frost caught his first whiff of ether off the silk pocket-handkerchief of Dr William Morton less than a century and a half ago!

8

Curious Arts

The identity and precise mechanism of the very first pain-killer lie buried in the morass of unrecorded history. It may have been a herb, innocently mashed and swallowed by some low-browed, voracious progenitor of man; or perhaps a club, swung out of pity; or maybe it was hypnotism (did not God put Adam into a deep sleep?).

Whatever the nature of the first, a wide variety of bizarre methods of killing pain have been used ever since over the ages. We know that the Babylonians and Assyrians employed more than 250 medicinal agents and that, included among these, were opium, hyoscyamus and hellebore. But administration of a drug, it was believed, had to be accompanied by the incantations of a priestly physician to be effective, and if the patient died, the 'doctor' was likely to have his fingers chopped off.

The Role of Magic

The ancient Egyptians were no more able to disentangle skills of pharmacy and medicine from magic and religion. The Eye of Horus, worn as an amulet strapped to the wrist or ankle, became a great pain-reliever and healing agent (Horus was a child-god), along with the eye of the newt and 'unicorn powders'.

The Egyptians also used pressure on nerves to prevent pain during surgery. Carvings on door-posts found in Egypt, dating back to 2500 BC, depict an operation in which one surgeon is squeezing the arm of the patient while another is operating on it. Later, this technique was extended to the throat: pressure was applied to the carotid arteries in the neck until the patient became unconscious; surgery was then performed, if possible, before consciousness returned.

By trial and error, repetitive accidents, and dimly perceived and often spurious relationships of cause and effect, the list of analgesic methods grew. But – since nobody knew what the inside of the body was really like, nor how it functioned – the physicians of antiquity were able to surround themselves with mystery. Indeed, one king of Egypt appointed his personal physician – a vizier known as Imhotep – to the status of God of Medicine!

The Greeks tried to sort out true efficacy from sorcery, but were only partially successful: Gods were still more powerful than drugs.

The Arabs, after the fall of Rome, succeeded in establishing pharmacy as a science, and stocked 'apothecaries' shops' with hundreds of exotic jars containing oils, powders, minerals, leaves, seeds and roots; but patients went on screaming in pain.

Galen, the Greek-born Roman physician of the second century AD gave considerable thought to the use of opium, hyoscyamus, hellebore and colocynth, obtaining his supplies from all over the world. But when the Roman Empire fell and the Goths, Huns and Vandals took over, medical practice in the West went into a decline, and superstition and magic were again left to fill the vacuum of ignorance.

Even under early Christianity, saints and holy relics were considered to be more potent then medicines, and the philosophy that it was good for the soul if the body had to endure pain was common dogma. Medicine in the Middle Ages has been described as a 'mish-mash of religion, magic and empirically acquired ideas and practices', and it was just that. But as the centuries passed, so patients began crying out for methods more effective than the prayers and incantations then offered to them.

The Soporific Lettuce

Monks began cultivating plants with pain-killing properties in their herb gardens, and administered them through the monastery hospitals to which the outside sick were admitted. Amongst these was the common lettuce, whose bitter, milky juice (*lactucarium*) had a sleep-inducing effect. Indeed, after the death of Adonis, Venus is said to have thrown herself 'upon a bed of lettuces, to lull her grief and repress her desires', and even as recently as 1909, Beatrix Potter was perpetuating the idea – in *Flopsy Bunnies* – that 'eating too much lettuce is soporific.' Galen, too, recorded that when he liberally ate of lettuce, a soothing slumber overtook him.

The Sleeping Sponge

But the favourite soporific anaesthetic of the Middle Ages was the sleeping sponge – *spongia somnifera* – a sea-sponge saturated with the mixed juices of plants, introduced in the ninth century. Its fumes were inhaled by the patient before surgery, and were supposed to render him insensible to pain. Yet surgeons who used it still insisted on tying down their patients with three straps: one across the chest, one encompassing the thighs and the third around the ankles.

Hugh de Lucca, the most renowned surgeon of the thirteenth century, provided the classic recipe for the sleeping sponge: a mixture of opium, mulberry juice, hyoscyamus, hemlock, mandragora, wood-ivy, apple-juice and the seeds of dock and ivy, all boiled together for one day. It was still in use in the sixteenth century when Valerius Cordus discovered 'sweet vitriol' (subsequently called ether) by distilling 'very biting wine', or alcohol with sulphuric acid.

'Sweet Vitriol'

Paracelsus, who gloried in calling his fellow-men in medicine liars, cheats, murders and ignoramuses, had this to say of 'sweet vitriol':

> The following should be noted here with regard to this sulfur; that of all things extracted from vitriol it is most remarkable because it is stable. And besides, it has associated with it such a sweetness that it is taken even by chickens, and they fall asleep from it for a while but awaken later without harm. On this sulfur no other judgement should be passed than that in diseases which need to be treated with anodynes it quiets all suffering without any harm, and relieves all pain, and quenches all fevers, and prevents complications in an illness.

It is, perhaps, extraordinary that 300 years were to elapse before Paracelsus's observation was put into clinical practice.

Pressure on nerves

However, uncertainty over the potency of narcotics, especially when mixed with wine, led to a gradual mistrust of this kind of preparation for surgery and, by the sixteenth century, physicians were turning once again to the ancient idea of nerve-trunk or arterial pressure. Valverde, the great Spanish surgeon of the Renaissance period, recorded in 1546:

> The carotids or *soporales*, that is, sleep-producing arteries, are so named because when they are pressed upon or closed in any way we soon go to sleep. This experiment I saw performed by Realdo Colombo in 1544 in Pisa on a young man in the presence of a number of gentlemen, with no less fear on their part than amusement on ours, we giving them to understand that it was done by sorcery.

Two centuries later, Benjamin Bell was recommending, in his *System of Surgery*:

> The pain induced by operation may be lessened in different ways; by diminishing the sensibility of the system; and by compressing the nerves that supply the parts upon which the operation is to be performed. . . . It has long been known that the sensibility of any part may not only be lessened, but even altogether suspended, by compressing the nerves that supply it; and accordingly, in amputating limbs, patients frequently desire the tourniquet to be firmly screwed, from finding that it tends to diminish the pain of operation.

A hideous armoury of clamps was devised for compressing limbs, before the practice went into decline and surgeons fell back on an old stand-by: alcohol.

Alcohol

Gin, rum, whisky: each has played a notable part in the battle against pain. Often, herbs were added to the alcohol. 'If it is desirable to get the person unconscious quickly,' wrote Avicenna in the eleventh century, 'add sweet-smelling moss or aloes-wood to the wine. If it is desirable to procure a deeply-unconscious state, so as to enable the pain to be borne, which is involved in painful applications to a member, place darnel-water into the wine.'

Henbane and mandragora were made into wines; Pliny had reported centuries previously that 'administered in doses proportioned to the strength of the patient, the juice of mandragora has a narcotic effect . . . it is given, too, for injuries inflicted by serpents and before incisions or punctures made in the body, in order to ensure insensibility to pain.'

Even as recently as 1973, a police surgeon reported in the journal *General Practitioner*:

> Alcohol has long been regarded by the medical profession as a useful drug. Its use as a cardiac stimulant, nervous-system depressant, and even as an antiseptic, is still fashionable. However, as an anaesthetic it has had to give way to more·modern drugs, but its basic potential for anaesthesia was illustrated this morning.
>
> At about half-past seven, I was called to the police station to see a male prisoner of twenty-six who complained of severe pain in the region of his right ankle. This man was seen

staggering in the road last night while drunk, and was arrested as much for his own sake as for any violation of the law. The station sergeant told me that even *he* thought there was something wrong with the man's ankle. He was dead right!

The whole ankle was grossly swollen, the slightest movement causing the man severe pain. The skin was badly discoloured, although there was no actual break of the surface. My patient told me that he thought he might have been run over by a van last night, but didn't really remember.

I was not too surprised, when I popped into the casualty department of the local hospital this afternoon, to be shown the X-rays of a second degree Pott's fracture. Looking back, it would appear that his alcohol intake had produced anaesthesia for at least six hours.

Alcohol is still given as a pain-killer in hospitals today, usually to terminal cancer patients and generally mixed with a powerful narcotic such as cocaine.

The sixteenth to eighteenth centuries were a wilderness, in so far as attempts to relieve or prevent pain were concerned. No matter how rich you were, nothing seemed to work. Consider this description by Sir Arthur Bryant, in *King Charles II* (Collins), of the last hours of the monarch, in 1685:

> An ever-growing number of physicians cupped, blistered, purged and scarified the King's tortured body. Three things only they denied him: light, rest and privacy; nothing else was left untried. As evening came on, they prepared against the night a whole army of violent remedies – scarcely a quarter passed but the remedies were applied – purges forced down the mouth, sneezing powders to the nose, burning plasters to the feet, thighs and arms, shoulders and head.

Often, the remedies were worse than the pain. Dr Victor Robinson, in *Victory over Pain* (H. K. Lewis & Co.), gives this description of surgery at the time:

> The patients were few in number, for the fear of pain was a deterrent equally as strong as the fear of possible accidents or of fatal errors by the surgeon. Many preferred to die rather than endure the exquisite agony which was in store for them. Once

brought to the table, they responded to the ordeal in various ways. Some struggled and screamed without remission, begging the surgeon to leave off or to make haste; some, usually the feeblest, fell into a trance-like state, which favoured the progress of the operation but gave little promise of survival; some bravely made no sign of suffering at all. Some cursed, some prayed.

Two centuries later, things were little better. Here is an extract from a grateful patient to Professor James Young Simpson, immediately after the discovery of anaesthesia:

Before the days of anaesthesia, a patient on the eve of his operation felt like a criminal who had been condemned to death and was now awaiting execution. He counted the days to the appointed time. He counted the hours on this last day and listened for the sound of the doctor's carriage. He anxiously followed his progress ringing the bell, setting foot on the stairs, entering his room, unpacking his instruments, saying a few serious words and making his last preparations. Then it was all up with his self-control. He rebelled against the necessity, insisted on being tied or held, in order to deliver himself helpless to the dreaded knife.

Military men, on the other hand, seemed to bear their pain stoically – perhaps because they knew that, to the civilian population, a wound was a badge of courage. David Howarth gives this account of surgery at the time of the battle of Waterloo in *Waterloo – A Near-Run Thing* (Collins):

A British surgeon carried his own outfit of knives, scalpels, saws, spare blades for the saws, tourniquets, forceps and strops to sharpen the knives on. These were fitted in a wooden case lined with plush, and kept bright with linseed oil. Beyond this, a recommended list of necessities was the following: lint, surgeon's tow, sponges, linen, both loose and in rollers, silk and wax for ligatures, whalebone splints, pins, tape, thread, needles, adhesive plaster ready-coated, opium, both solid and in tincture, submuriate of mercury, antimonials, sulphate of magnesia, volatile alkali, oil of turpentine, wax candles, phosphoric matches, and a canteen of good wine or spirits diluted; for as a medical handbook said, 'Many men sink beyond recovery for want of a timely cordial before, during and after operations.'

Soldiers at least knew what to expect if they were wounded and reached the surgeons alive; there was nothing esoteric or complex in their treatment. For chest or abdominal wounds, nothing could be done except plaster or stitch the external wound together and wait and see what happened. Extensive abdominal operations had been performed by civil surgeons, but the chance of survival was so small that no surgeon in battle would think of wasting time on them. For legs or arms, however, there was a ready remedy: cut them off. Soldiers believed that surgeons lopped off arms and legs by the cartload to save themselves trouble. There was some truth in that. It did save trouble, both for the surgeons and the patients. . . .

The most surprising thing to the modern mind is that men would submit to the probing, stitching, cutting and sawing, without any kind of anaesthetic, yet without any overwhelming dread. The wine and diluted spirits the surgeons carried were given, in moderate doses, to strengthen the patients, not to make them insensible; the opiates were to rest them after the operation, not before. One surgeon, discussing broken bones, wrote that 'after the action of Waterloo, the excruciating torture brought on by the slightest attempt at setting the limbs was in some instances very remarkable'.

Men in those days, one must suppose, were not less sensitive to pain than they are now. But pain was familiar, in themselves and others. So they were less afraid of it than later generations brought up with anaesthetics; and perhaps the fear of pain is exaggerated now, in people who have never had a serious pain and know it can be avoided. Besides that, it was part of a soldier's code to go through an amputation with an air of unconcern. A French prisoner who picked up his sawn-off leg and threw it into the air shouting 'Vive l'Empéreur' was thought eccentric by the British who happened to see. But everyone admired an officer at Mont St Jean who refused to be helped from the table when his leg had been cut off, but jumped down and hopped unaided to the cart that was waiting to take him to Brussels.

The relief of pain remained in the hands of the apothecary, or in the doubtful solace of the bottle. The London drug-trade, which had remained under the control of grocers until 1617, still offered as late as 1820 such repulsive preparations as 'live spiders rolled in butter', 'powdered mummy', 'ant eggs', the feathers of partridges and 'the eyes of crabs'. Quacks handed out powdered sapphire for strengthening vision, thistles for healing cuts, pulverized emeralds for sexual troubles, and gold flakes in wine to promote longevity.

Doctors had to combat not only quacks but formidable amateur competition as well. Unqualified medical advice was dispensed from mouth to mouth, and it was not beneath the clergy from time to time to step in with some dynamic prescription. Bishop George Berkeley, for example, was one who preached the virtues of 'tar-water' as a panacea for all ills: 'Stir a quart of tar into a gallon of water, let it settle for forty-eight hours, pour off the clear water, drink it and be cured of what ails you.'

It was into such a climate of intrigue and suspicion that an affluent Austrian mystic came upon the scene in 1774, with a new idea: that the lodestone could influence pain and disease in the body. His name: Franz Anton Mesmer.

Mesmerism

Franz Anton Mesmer was a gentleman of means. Born of affluent parents, he dallied first with the Church, then with the Law and finally, in 1766, qualified in medicine. He took a keen interest in all new developments in the sciences and the arts, patronized concerts, conducted discussions about abstract philosophy, and threw open his house in Vienna to his many friends, to whom he was both a genial and generous host. Mozart was amongst his closest companions, as was the then Professor of Astronomy at the University of Vienna, a Jesuit with the name of Pater Hell.

It was through the latter that Mesmer became interested in the mysterious power of the lodestone. What made it behave as it did? Whence came its power to attract and repel? Might it not be able to influence more than just little pieces of iron?

Mindful of the writings of Paracelsus – or rather of those parts suggested that the stars might influence the health and general condition of humans by way of a subtle and invisible fluid – Mesmer propounded a different kind of fluid: 'magnetic fluid'. It was, he suggested, susceptible to the power of the lodestone. Mesmer made the magnet a symbol of healing. If two magnets were placed on the body of a sick person, 'animal magnetism' would flow through that body and cure it of its ills.

He began to experiment. He tried his 'cure' on a wide variety of conditions, from stomach-ache to deafness, from earache to blindness or even paralysis. So successful was his treatment that news of it spread like wildfire through Vienna. The council of the Augsburg Academy issued a report in 1776 which stated: 'What Dr Mesmer has achieved in the way of curing the most diverse maladies leads us to suppose that he has discovered one of Nature's mysterious motive energies.' But his medical colleagues in Vienna spurned him. 'Animal magnetism' became a joke.

Rebuffed, Mesmer abandoned Vienna for Paris, and Paris was receptive. The smell of Revolution was in the air. Mysticism was in vogue. The rich craved new thrills, the poor miracles. Anyone with mystical powers was welcome in the salons where the activities of Cagliostro and Madame Bontemps had become legend. The flamboyant Mesmer, with his magnets, was an immediate success.

'Animal magnetism', which by now had extended its reputation not only to cure ailments but to anaesthetize against pain, became such a hot topic that duels were even arranged between its supporters and its opponents. Marie Antoinette became a protagonist. Nobility flocked for treatment; indeed, so many wanted a session with Mesmer that he had to give up treating patients individually and, instead, treated them in groups.

He had ceased actually pressing magnets against the skins of patients; instead, he took a metal rod, rubbed a magnet along it and then pointed the rod at the assembled group. Later, he elaborated by dressing in a long silk robe, dimming the lights and playing soft music during his treatment sessions. Later still, he dispensed with the rod and used just his own hands, discovering that the effect was just as dramatic. Finally, he dispensed with the laying on of hands and merely *told* his patients that their pains would disappear, or that their maladies would improve. And frequently they did.

He invented a tub which could be sold for use by patients in their own homes. Each tub contained bottles of his special 'magnetic fluid', lined up in such a way that they pointed towards the centre, converging on a rod. From the rod extended wires which had to be placed over any parts of the patient's body in which pain could be felt or disease was suspected. He magnetized wash-basins (so that pain could be washed away), mirrors (so that patients would look better) and even whole houses.

For a while, he was the idol of Paris. He was offered a pension if he would reveal his 'secret', but turned it down, saying he wanted scientific recognition, not money. Eventually, Louis XVI appointed a commission of the Faculty of Medicine and the Académie des Sciences to investigate his 'animal magnetism'. Its members concluded that there was no evidence to justify his claims.

Mesmer was furious. But soon afterwards the Revolution broke out, and many of his 'patients' went to the guillotine. He fled to Vienna, where he was immediately arrested on suspicion of being a spy. However, he was eventually released and allowed to retire to his birthplace – Meersburg – where ultimately, in 1815, he died. Mesmer was a charlatan in that his methods were unscientific; it was not the magnetism of the lodestone which did the trick but the magnetism of his own personality. He used, albeit unwittingly, hypnotism.

This was proved shortly before his death by one of his followers in Paris, Count Maxime de Puysegur. It had been a favourite gimmick of Mesmer that he could improve the vitality of trees, by stroking them with a magnet. One day, de Puysegur tied a shepherd to one of these 'mesmerized' trees in order to cure his pain. The Count gently waved his hands in front of his eyes, murmuring soothing words, only to discover that the old man immediately went into a trance. He instructed him to untie himself, which he did, and then ordered him to weave a complicated path through the garden – which again he did, like an automaton. The shepherd was oblivious to all but the Count's commands until told to wake up.

By 1830, many Parisian physicians were using hypnotism as a therapeutic agent, and the practice spread to Britain. One of those impressed by it was.John Elliotson, then first Professor of Medicine at the new University of London. Elliotson gave demonstrations of mesmerism to, amongst others, the novelists Dickens and Thackeray, in which he sat his patient in a darkened room, passed his hands over him and breathed on the crown of his head. An hour or so later, when the patient's trance had deepened, he would operate on him painlessly.

Elliotson's practices became the subject of such controversy that eventually the Council of University College, London passed a resolution forbidding him from using the technique within the hospital. He resigned, practised privately, lived to see others copy his technique in America and India – indeed, several thousand operations were performed painlessly on 'mesmerized' patients – before retiring into comparative obscurity.

Eventually, in March 1850, a London Mesmeric Infirmary was set up at 9 Bedford Square; others were set up in Bristol, Exeter and Dublin. But all were eclipsed before long by the advent of ether and chloroform.

Hypnotism

The year was 1838. The place: Wellow District Hospital, Nottinghamshire. The patient was a 42-year-old labourer, James Wombell, who for five years had suffered from a neglected disease of the left knee. Even the slightest movement of the joint caused him such pain that the only way he could find any comfort was to sit up in bed.

Even then, the lightest contact with the bedclothes was agonizing.

Squire Ward, the surgeon consulted over the case, decided that the best way to end the man's misery would be to amputate the limb from above the knee. Accordingly, Wombell was put to sleep, breathing quietly and regularly during the thirty-minute operation; shortly afterwards he was awakened with a draught of sal volatile, and the next day was heard singing. The anaesthetist in the case was not, however, a medical practitioner but a barrister of the Middle Temple, and the method he used to tranquillize his patient was nothing other than hypnotic suggestion.

Hypnotism is still practised in medicine and dentistry today. The British Society of Medical and Dental Hypnosis, set up in the early 1950s, has more than 600 members, its American counterpart – the Society of Clinical Hypnosis – twice as many. The advantage of using hypnosis to relieve or prevent pain is that it is safe and non-toxic. Unfortunately, it is not always effective. Only a proportion of people are susceptible enough for it to remove pain. The patient's attention has to be fixed so that he or she becomes hyper-suggestible, willing to accept illogical ideas from the hypnotist. Many cannot concentrate hard enough or are unwilling for this to happen.

Dentists who practise hypnosis report that about 35 per cent of patients can be sufficiently hypnotized to feel numbness enough to make the injection of a needle painless. Also, hypnotism will frequently allay alarm at the prospect of an extraction or similar operation. But deep hypnosis, so that the patient does not even need an anaesthetic, is only possible in between 10 and 20 per cent of cases. In medicine, Dr L. Goldie reported that hypnosis was the only anaesthetic needed by some patients in setting fractured bones and dislocated joints at the casualty department of Maudsley Hospital while he was à registrar there. Skin-stitches can similarly be inserted in susceptible patients. Moreover, a medium trance-state has repeatedly been proved to take the pain out of daunting surgical dressings, repeated lumbar punctures and tapping the nasal sinuses.

A Finnish doctor has used hypnosis to relieve headache and vertigo in patients who suffered from these conditions several years after skull injuries. Dr Claes Cedercreutz, of the Regional Hospital in Hamina, says that since 1969 he has treated 120 patients by hypnosis after no satisfactory treatment was found for their condition. 43 had headaches, 72 had headaches and vertigo, and 5 vertigo alone. Following hypnotherapy, 57 patients were symptom-free and there were ameliorated symptoms in another 24.

The same doctor has used hypnosis for the treatment of 'phantom limb' pain; he made it disappear in 22 out of 100 cases and it became less severe in a further 13. And, in a report to the *International Journal of Clinical Experimental Hypnosis* (vol. 9, no. 3), he claims that he has eliminated the pain of osteo-arthritis, sciatica, post-operative scars, lung cancer and spasms of the blood-vessels, intestine, ureters and bladder in suitable patients, including several who had undergone repeated surgery without obtaining any relief. He adds: 'I believe that hypnosis is a valuable and far too seldom employed weapon for combating pain. The surgical staff of every large hospital should include a hypnotist. With his aid, it would be possible in 25 per cent of cases to make pain disappear without an operation and this would be of great benefit.'

Dr Paul Van Dyke of Suffern, New York, goes further: 'I believe that it is universally accepted by all those that are acquainted with it that hypnosis can benefit every surgical patient,' he writes. 'Its value to the patient is determined by the way it is used by the operator; and the way it is used by the operator is dependent on his training and skill and his goals in using hypnosis.'

In a report to the *American Journal of Clinical Hypnosis* (April 1970), Dr Van Dyke gives an interesting account of the use of hypnosis on a girl of six.

I had operated on her for acute purulent appendicitis with peritonitis. At the time of her first post-operative dressing, I induced a trance-state by using the TV-game method. She closed her eyes, pretended she was at home and was permitted to look at any program she wished. She reached out with her hand and turned on the TV. While the picture tube was warming up, I suggested that she relax in her favourite TV viewing-chair and when the tube finally lit up she could let me know by just moving her index-finger. When I received her signal, I started changing her dressing, removing the saturated gauze, replacing it with dry gauze, and shortening her drain a bit. As is usual in any TV show, the program was interrupted by commercials. I told her to indicate to me by moving the same finger when the commercial began. When she so indicated, I used this commercial time to present a commercial of my own.

I complimented her on her ability to relax and to see so well the TV show that she chose and to enjoy it so much; and told her that each time I asked her to play this game she could do it better and better, and enjoy it more and more. At the end of the commercial her program resumed, and I resumed my activity with her dressing. Her trance-state was sufficiently deep, and she enjoyed it so much, that she paid no attention at all to my activities regarding her dressing and her drain. A severe adhesive-tape reaction complicated her healing. This was treated by means of benzine, alcohol, and the application of compound tincture of benzion; and she presented no evidence of the perception of any pain or discomfort at any time. Ordinarily a situation like this – a draining abdominal wound in a child, on which is superimposed a contact dermatitis of a large area of skin – is apt to present a very trying prospect to the patient, and also to the attending surgeon. Hypnosis took care of the pain.

In a controlled clinical trial at Cardiff Maternity Hospital, obstetrician John Hughes found that hypnosis reduced the duration of labour from an average of 11 ½ hours to 6 ½ hours, and that whereas 67 per cent of mothers receiving ordinary care needed strong, pain-killing drugs, only 40 per cent did under hypnosis.

Dr Vincent Cangello of Oakland, California uses hypnosis for the treatment of cancer pains. In a report on twenty-two cases (*International Journal of Clinical Experimental Hypnosis*, vol. 9, no. 1) he states that thirteen requested less narcotics after hypnosis. He concludes:

This form of management should be given a trial for the relief of pain in malignant disease before resorting to either chemical rhizotomy or surgical tractotomy, since it is relatively simple to perform, has virtually no rate of complication or morbidity, is successful in a satisfactory proportion of the cases, and is not unduly time-consuming.

How then can hypnosis affect sensibility to pain? One theory put forward recently suggests that the 'gate control' mechanism of the spinal cord (see Chapter 2) can be activated by hypnosis so that it cuts out local reflexes.

In a paper to *Psychological Review* (vol. 80, no. 5) in 1973, Dr Ernest Hilgard of the Department of Psychology, Stanford University describes experiments in which hypnosis was used on volunteers to block the pain brought on by exercising a limb after its blood-supply had been cut off by a tourniquet:

In some of these experiments, suggested hypnotic analgesia has appeared to reduce both heart-rate and blood-pressure below the levels found in the normal non-hypnotic condition. If these results are substantiated, they can be interpreted as evidence that local reflexes can be abolished by a gate control mechanism activated hypnotically, as suggested by Wall. Ischemic pain, by contrast with cold, may be mediated almost exclusively by the two pain mechanisms that interact at the dorsal horn level.

Dr Hilgard sums up:

> Pain reduction through hypnosis has baffled scientists ever
> since its successful use in major surgery in the early nineteenth
> century. The search for more satisfactory explanations might
> have continued except that the development of chloroform and
> ether brought an early end to the use of hypnosis for the
> purpose of general anaesthesia. This was not actually quite the
> end, however, for hypnosis has been used for pain reduction to
> some extent ever since, and more recently there has been an
> upsurge of its use in obstetrics, in the relief of painful burns, in
> dental extractions, in terminal cancer, and (to a lesser extent) in
> a variety of surgical operations. . . . While there are always
> some doubting Thomases, the evidence is overwhelming that
> some patients through hypnotic suggestion alone can endure
> normally painful experiences of stress without feeling any pain
> whatsoever.

Auto-suggestion and Yoga

In parts of the Deccan plateau in India, it is still possible to meet
members of a tribe known as the Ras Phasé Pardhi. The Pardhi are
nomadic and are accompanied on their travels by a few scrawny
cattle; their main occupation is theft.

They cling to a number of ancient rituals, mostly religious, including a fertility dance whose climax is for the dancer to plunge his hand
into a cauldron of boiling oil. He apparently feels nothing. Another
Pardhi custom is for a person accused of a crime to demonstrate his
innocence by walking a fixed number of paces whilst carrying a piece
of red-hot iron.

Elsewhere on the Deccan plateau, in a few remote villages, sharp
hooks are still clawed into living flesh in preparation for the ancient
'swinging' ritual (which is actually a celebration). One eyewitness
who returned from India recently, gave me this description:

> In this village the two swinging posts are set up in a cart that is
> used only on this one day of the year. Nowadays, the cele-
> brant's weight is no longer borne by the hooks throughout the
> ceremony. Between swings, he sits more or less comfortably
> astride a bar suspended from a crossbeam that is balanced
> between the two uprights. A new crossbeam is ceremonially
> cut each year, in a jungle some forty miles from the village, for
> this purpose. The celebrant is led to the local temple. There
> he is ritually bathed, declared deva (temporarily divine) and

dressed in a special costume (a red turban and red silk trousers) that leaves him naked from the waist up.

The celebrant now goes to the site of the village's annual hoil (spring festival) bonfire. He stands on the fire's ashes as the village carpenter thrusts the two steel hooks into the small of his back. Every man in the village crowds around to watch the operation. The celebrant is then decked with garlands and led to a nearby field. There the bagad cart, drawn by a pair of bullocks, is waiting. A rope that is attached to each hook is looped behind the celebrant's back and tied to the crossbeam, which rests on the two bagad uprights. The celebrant individually blesses each child born since the last hook-swinging; when this has been done, he makes his first swing suspended by the hooks. A cheer goes up, the god-elect nimbly climbs astride his resting bar and the cart jolts off across the fields.

At prescribed points along the route, the cart stops and the celebrant descends from the bar to make a predetermined number of swings. After all the village's fields have been blessed in this manner, the procession continues through the fields of a neighbouring village to the place where the god Mhatoba's temple stands. The people have gathered from miles around. A number of goats are now sacrificed, the order of their slaughter being established by the rank of the clan offering the sacrifice.

When the sacrifices are over, the hook-ropes are untied from the bagad beam and the god-elect climbs down from his bar. He enters the temple, the hooks are removed, and his wounds are anointed with ashes from Mhatoba's sacred fire. Once this is done, the god-elect reverts to human status. During the ceremony that I observed, the celebrant was in a state of exaltation and showed no trace of pain. Although he received no medical treatment other than the application of wood-ash, two weeks later the marks on his back were scarcely visible.

Such feats of mind over matter are not uncommon in a country where Yoga is widely practised. But some of the demonstrations ascribed to yogis are not demonstrations of yoga at all, according to Abdulhusein Dalai and Dr Theodore Barber, two American research workers who investigated a number of so-called 'yogic feats' in 1969. 'A common belief is that yogis are able to lie on a bed of nails and to thrust metal spikes into their flesh,' they wrote in the *American Journal of Clinical Hypnosis* (January 1969),

However, the first author, during his seven years' training in yoga, did not hear of any practitioner who claimed to be able to perform such feats. Rather, they are performed by a small number of fakirs and dervishes (religious mendicants) who are often confused with yogis. Although Wenger and Bagchi (1961) found no individuals in India 'who stuck needles into their bodies', they found one person who lay on beds of nails. Wenger and Bagchi noted that 'For the latter the task was easy. By practice he had learned to relax the muscles of the back, and the nails were close together and not very sharp.' It should also be noted that the apparent 'analgesia' or the stoicism may at times be due to the fact that some of these individuals who lie on nails are addicted to hashish or opium (Rawcliffe, 1959). When the nails are not blunt and when no drugs are taken, the performance demonstrates a not too unusual ability to tolerate a certain amount of pain.

As a boy in India, I recall seeing a man skip across a shallow pit containing smoking-hot stones. But as the two American researchers point out:

The feat of fire-walking also takes on a somewhat different appearance in the light of the following observations: 'In south India and in other locations it [fire-walking] seems to be a common practice in connection with religious or other celebrations. We are informed, however, that the coals are well covered with ashes and that the 'walk' is more like a 'run'. Moreover, the participants are not yogis: they are the young men of the villages. And, since they have seldom or never worn shoes, the epidermis of the soles of their feet is reported to us as being ⅛ to ¼ inch in thickness. There may be fire-walkers with tender feet, but we have not seen them or heard about them in India' [Wenger and Bagchi, 1961].

Apparently, no case of fire-walking by a yogi has as yet been documented, whereas numerous non-yogis have rather easily performed the 'feat'. Among the latter is a British university student who walked in bare feet with perfect safety across a twelve-foot trench with a surface temperature of 800°C.

There was not the slightest trace of blistering . . . each foot was in contact with the embers for not more than about a third of a second. This time-factor (plus confidence and a steady, deliberate placing of the feet) is the secret of fire-walking. The low thermal conductivity of the wood-ash may be a contributory factor. We received no evidence that 'faith' or a specially induced mental state played any part in the performance.

The fire-walking feat as also been performed before competent observers in the United States by Coe, a chemist living in Florida, in 1957. With eight steps he crossed bare-footed a fourteen-foot pit of red-hot coals without suffering pain or forming blisters. After reviewing the literature of physics and chemistry to discover possible principles that might be involved, he proffered the following hypothesis: 'First there is natural moisture present on the surface of the skin. Under intense heat, the skin sweats and the moisture, which enters the spheroidal state, is converted to vapor which occupies 22.4 molar volumes of the original moisture. This is why a microscopically thin layer of moisture can be a protection. . . . The hotter the object, the longer the spheroidal state is maintained, and the greater the protection afforded by the cushion of vapor.' Whether or not Coe's hypothesis accounts for the phenomenon can be determined in further research.

Frederick Prescott, in his book *The Control of Pain* (Hodder & Stoughton Educational) relates:

There are travellers' stories of ceremonies in Tibet in which the participants gather in a circle, and dance to the accompaniment of chants until they work themselves into a hypnotic frenzy. While they are in a trance-like state, the dancers pass needles through their cheeks and the fleshy parts of their bodies without flinching and without causing bleeding. No pain is felt in this trance-like state. The Tibetan mystics concentrate on some thought so that they become insensitive to pain. . . . Witches, who were persecuted as late as the beginning of the eighteenth century, were said to have areas on their body insensitive to pain. These were searched for with great care by sticking needles all over the naked body of the victim. If an anaesthetic spot, the so-called devil's mark, were found, this was diagnostic of a witch. Witches were also accused of preventing pain at childbirth, which they did by getting the expectant mother to stare intently at an object made of steel or iron for a long time.

The French author, Heuzé, reported in 1926 how he stuck hat-pins through his flesh without feeling pain. Such performances, he insisted, could be learned by most individuals who possess 'average patience and fortitude'.

This is certainly true of the Chinese.

Acupuncture

The ancient Chinese believed that the basis of all life is a force of energy called *Qi* (pronounced 'chee'), circulating around the body along channels called 'meridians'. The meridians are linked to the twelve major body-organs, to which they send branches; there is also a thirteenth meridian at the front of the body and a fourteenth at the back.

The flow of *Qi*, according to the Taoist philosophy in which the ancients believed, is under the control of 'yin' and 'yang', two universal opposites existing throughout Nature. Yin represents negative forces – darkness, passivity, cold, femininity, and so forth – while yang represents positives like heat, light, activity and masculinity. A healthy person, the Chinese believed, must maintain a precise balance between yin and yang; sickness results when an imbalance occurs. The Chinese taught that for the healthy state to exist there has to be a free and unimpeded flow of *Qi*. Any obstruction causes a deficiency in one part of the body with a corresponding excess in another. And the only way to correct an imbalance – when disease breaks out or the body is in pain – is to stimulate the flow of *Qi* at certain points along the meridians.

There are a thousand of these points, the so-called 'acupuncture' points. Their numbers vary along the different meridians – the heart meridian, for example, has only nine whereas the bladder meridian has sixty-seven and the liver twenty – but they each have a precise anatomical location and an identifying name and number (such as 'stomach 43').

What the acupuncturist does is to insert stainless steel or gold needles into some of these points, and either twirl or vibrate them. Some of the points are supposed to increase the flow of *Qi*, others to retard it. The acupuncturist follows a complex set of laws governing the relationship between the various body-organs when he inserts the needles, and may twirl several needles along several meridians simultaneously in order to alleviate pain or disease in one organ. He may also emplace them well away from the apparent location of the trouble. 'Stomach 43', for example, is situated above the division of the second and third toe, yet apparently relieves stomach-ache; 'liver 1' is also in the foot, yet influences the liver.

The Chinese have been using acupuncture (the word comes from the Latin 'acus' meaning a needle) for nearly 5,000 years. But it was only in the 1930s, when the Chinese Communists waged guerrilla war on the Nationalists, that it received its first official support. Faced with a desperate shortage of drugs and Western-trained doctors, Mao-Tse-Tung and his fellow guerrillas turned to the acupuncturists and herbalists. 'Chinese medicine and pharmacology are a great treasure-house,' declared Mao, 'and effort should be made to explore them and raise them to a higher level.' He decreed that acupuncture classes should be held in all provinces which came under Communist control.

Today, the Chinese use acupuncture to treat a whole range of conditions, from malaria to blindness and rheumatism to hypertension. Although claims of success have to be treated with caution because of the paucity of scientific literature coming out of China, according to one report all but 2 out of 280 cases of goitre were cured by acupuncture administered every other day for two weeks. According to another, 253 out of 526 polio victims treated at Peking Municipal Children's Hospital made complete recoveries. In 1970, the Chinese reported that more than 1,000 persons with serious eye-disorders were treated with acupuncture, and that nine out of ten showed improvement; a total of 111 persons blind for up to forty years regained their sight.

To date, more than 500,000 operations have been performed in the People's Republic of China since 1968 in which acupuncture was used as the main anaesthetic. Some of these have been watched by Western observers. One of these – Dr Michael de Bakey, the Texas heart surgeon – gave this description of an open-heart operation performed on a 21-year-old Chinaman in a Shanghai hospital:

> The young man lay supine on the operating table when I entered the operating theatre of the Third Municipal Hospital. He was awake, but so drowsy that I asked if he had received any drugs. The anaesthetist said that he had been given phenobarbitone, a sedative, and ten milligrammes of morphine, a narcotic pain-killer. Neither dose was strong enough to anaesthetize, but together they relaxed the patient and put him in a suggestible state.
>
> Now the acupuncturist began inserting various lengths of stainless steel needles at carefully selected points. Each needle had a wire finger-grip extending along all but about an inch of its shaft. The acupuncturist twirled the needles rapidly as he inserted them: four in the left ear, one each in the undersides of the forearms, another in each hand at the junction of thumb and forefinger.
>
> When they were in place, he attached an electric wire to each needle and connected them to a generator, which sent a pulsing current of about 120 cycles a minute to the eight points. The effect was visible in a spasmodic pulsing of the patient's hands.

In previous acupuncture operations, I had seen the needles electrified, but I had also seen them manipulated by hand, with the acupuncturist twirling the shafts while at the same time raising and plunging the needles up and down through the tissue beneath the skin. Both approaches seemed to provide about the same outcome for the patient. And it didn't seem to make a great deal of difference where the needles were inserted. In one operation, for example, just a single needle was inserted in the top of the forearm. For the same type of operation in another hospital, the needle was sunk into the underside of the forearm. In another, it was inserted in an ear.

Today, the needles took effect in about ten minutes. But before the chief surgeon reached for his scalpel, he injected a local anaesthetic into the skin-tissues around the young man's breastbone. Other members of the surgical team said later that such locals were often used, because otherwise patients felt the pain of the first surgical incision in their skin. This was the only time I saw a local used before the initial incision.

The surgeon began tracing an incision along the length of the breastbone with his scalpel. I watched the patient's face carefully. He never flinched. Nor did he appear to be the least bit concerned when his breastbone was partially split with hammer and chisel, a rather rough procedure which shakes the patient severely.

So, how does acupuncture work? It would appear that the calm behaviour of the patients has a psychological rather than physiological explanation, and is perhaps a form of self-hypnosis. But another American observer who visited Shanghai, Dr Jack Geiger, concluded: 'The anaesthetic effect is not due to any kind of hypnosis, unless one is willing to accept the unlikely proposition that horses, mules, cats, rats, rabbits, and human infants are susceptible to hypnosis, whether by standard techniques or by acupuncture needling.'

In a report to *World Medicine* (August 1973), Dr Geiger revealed some of the Chinese' own conclusions:

The Chinese have found that acupuncture changes the patient's perception of both the intensity and quality of pain by specific blocking actions at two and perhaps three levels of the central nervous system, without the cortical depression and alteration in consciousness that accompanies traditional chemical anaesthesia. The effect of acupuncture needling, they believe, is on the proprioceptors: muscle spindles and related stretch and pressure receptors. The vigorous neurological discharge over proprioceptive pathways induced by acupuncture needles acts, by a kind of competitive ·inhibition, to block pain-impulses carried over cutaneous nerves and other afferent pain-fibres.

The blocking action, presumably mediated by internuncial neurones, occurs in the spinal cord's posterior horn and in at least two nuclei in the thalamus long known to be associated with transmission of pain-impulses from spinal cord to cerebral cortex. It is affected by the general level of CNS excitability and thus by cortical activity.

At least some of the most important of the traditional acupuncture-points have been shown to lie above particularly heavy concentrations of proprioceptors in muscle and tendon tissue. Vigorous and prolonged massage and deep pressure on proprioceptors – in areas in which this is anatomically possible, such as the traditional Ho-ku acupuncture point on the dorsal aspect of the hand between the bases of the thumb and index-finger – will induce surgical anaesthesia (sufficient, for example, to perform a thyroidectomy) without the use of acupuncture needles. Presumably, then, either needling or deep massage can stimulate the necessary neurological discharge along proprioceptive pathways.

Inhibition or blocking of pain-impulses in the spinal cord, and in thalamic nuclei, has been demonstrated repeatedly under controlled experimental conditions by classic neurobiological techniques, including oscilloscopic recordings of microelectrodes inserted in single axons, myographic recording of the contractions of myofibrils, and quantitative measurement of responses to standardized pain stimuli in experimental animals before, during, and after acupuncture needling.

But after experiments on standard acupuncture sites in the arms of volunteers, two New York research workers – W. Crawford Clark and J. C. Yang – concluded that acupuncture anaesthesia worked as a result of *expectation* on the part of the patient and not because of any blocking of the nerves. 'Pain', they point out (*Science*, vol. 184), 'consists of two parts: the physiological sensory perception and the psychological appreciation. It has been shown that when subjects are given placebos in places of powerful analgesics, the threshold at which pain – say, from a heat source – is felt increases. Nevertheless, the sensory perception remains the same. And so it is with acupuncture.' In other words, people who do not feel pain after acupuncture are *willing* themselves not to feel it, blocking it from their minds.

Whatever the explanation, more and more Western doctors are using acupuncture. One estimate puts the total at 15,000 in Britain and Europe, and several hundred in the US; in France and the Soviet Union it is even possible to have acupuncture on the health service. One doctor I know in North London uses it to treat chronic cases of migraine, duodenal ulcer, fibrositis, lumbago, sciatica, neuralgia, asthma and acne. And a survey of more than 600 consecutive cases treated by acupuncture, by 10 doctors in various parts of Britain, yielded the following results:

Condition treated	No. of Patients	Cured or much improved (%)	Slightly improved (%)	No change (%)
Migraine	119	56	20	24
Arthritis (all groups)	196	25	50	25
Rheumatic conditions	95	33	57	10
Asthma	57	50	25	25
Vasomotor rhinitis and hay fever	51	40	40	20
Dysmenorrhoea	26	50	16	34
Peptic ulcer and indigestion	41	30	35	35
General psychiatric	30	30	35	35
Impotence and frigidity	27	25	25	50
Total	642	37	33	30

(Proceedings of the Royal Society of Medicine, May 1973)

The truth about the efficacy of acupuncture probably lies somewhere between the most enthusiastic claims and the harshest criticism. As Dr Paul Dudley White, the American physician, puts it: 'If it were the world's best technique, we'd all be using it; if it were useless, it would have been dropped thousands of years ago. There's something in it, but it's difficult to say what.'

Other Chinese Treatments

Yin and yang are thought to have been the concepts of Fu Hsi, a Chinese emperor who lived around 3,000 BC. He was followed by another emperor, Shen Nung, who according to legend had a transparent stomach. This enabled him to observe the actions of poisons and their antidotes through his abdominal wall and, as a result, to build up a pharmacopoeia of therapeutic substances, including some to alleviate pain: poppy juice, for example, to soothe crying babies; chestnut to relieve piles; and sage to take soreness from throats. There were numerous other vegetable remedies – the sea-grape (whose alkaloid, Ephedrine, is still used in the treatment of asthma and allergies today), aconite, calamus, angelica, vetch, lotus, ginseng and ginger, to name but a few – together with some which smacked of the black arts: for example extract of donkey's skin; urine from a boy; sweat from a toad; and the flesh of snakes.

Another old Chinese method of treating pain was Moxa. Moxa was a burning therapy. It involved compressing the hairs of the plant artemesia (mugwort) into a wad which could be rolled into little cylinders of paper about the size of a cigarette. The roll was then set alight and held against the skin until a small burn appeared. The Chinese believed that the burning had to be done on special zones on the body to be effective, but they used it as a treatment for headache, toothache, migraine, gout, abdominal pain, colic and inflammatory conditions, as well as for diarrhoea, vertigo and nose-bleed. Moxa worked by counter-irritation: certain albuminous compounds in the tissues of the patient were released by the burning process and carried along by the bloodstream to act as a counter-irritant, so taking the patient's mind off the condition and allowing the body to reverse it. Use of the technique was revived in the early 1920s by a Berlin surgeon, August Bior, but it never really caught on.

Audio-analgesia

A more effective way of taking the patient's mind off pain is audio-analgesia. Audio-analgesia presents stereophonic, tape-recorded music combined with a 'white noise' generator which produces a sound rather like that of Niagara Falls; its purpose is to eliminate pain and discomfort during most dental procedures.

It was first introuded into dentistry in 1959 by two Boston dentists – Wallace Gardner and J. C. R. Licklider – who reported using it initially on 387 patients during cavity preparation, scaling and grinding operations, claiming 'it produced completely effective analgesia in 68 per cent'. Then they used it on 119 patients who needed extractions: 'In every instance, the patient was aware of the pressure and the pull, and in some instances moderate pain was reported, but in no instance was there severe pain or regret for not having used a conventional anaesthetic.'

In their first report in the *Journal of the American Dental Association* (vol. 59, December 1959), the two dentists give a lovely description of their first experiment with audio–analgesia on themselves. Licklider was the 'patient' while Gardner drilled out a large cavity:

Although both patient and dentist were at first incredulous, it was evident that the sound had a direct suppressive effect upon the pain.

The office secretary was immediately pressed into service as patient and observer. This young woman had a history of extreme fearfulness in the dental chair. She had never before had cavities prepared without a local anaesthetic or an analgesic. Nevertheless, she agreed to forgo the use of conventional agents. She put on the earphones, adjusted the volume of the masking sound and sat quietly through the preparation of three large cavities without appearing to experience any pain. At the end of the session, she reported that she had felt none.

Following this report, a piece of electronic equipment called 'The Audio Analgesiac' went into commercial production. Licklider gives this description of it in use:

> The patient wears earphones and controls his own acoustic stimulation through a control-box held in his lap. It has two control knobs, one for music and the other for a rushing, roaring sound derived from 'white noise'. At the beginning of the session, the patient selects the music he wants to hear – a stereophonic tape recording – and adjusts it to a volume suitable for ordinary listening. When the dentist starts to work, or when his work causes any discomfort, the patient turns up the volume of the music. As soon as there is a trace or forewarning of pain, the patient turns the noise knob. It controls the level of the rushing, roaring 'waterfall' sound. The overall sound-pressure of the noise may be set as high as 116 decibels above 0.0002 microbar.

The two dentists originally listed seven factors which, they considered, contributed to the pain-killing power of the technique:

1. The noise appears to directly suppress the pain caused by dental procedure.
2. The noise masks the sound of the dental drill, thereby removing a source of 'conditioned anxiety'.
3. Thus music, and the noise, which sounds like a waterfall, have a relaxing effect.
4. When both music and noise are presented, the music can be followed only through concentration, which distracts attention away from the dental operation.
5. Active participation gives the patient a feeling of control over a situation which formerly seemed completely out of his hands.
6. The dentist can judge the patient's state of anxiety or discomfort by noting whether the patient is using music or noise, and by observing the intensity of each signal.
7. Suggestion.

But they went further. They claimed that audio-analgesia directly acted on the nervous system at points where it came into contact with the auditory system; in other words, in several regions of the reticular formation of the brain and the thalamus.

Arguments broke out amongst research workers. Dr Jack Howitt in Rochester, New York, conducted experiments on 138 children to try to find out which components in audio-analgesia were really having an effect. He reported that the effect was largely due to suggestion, and that the same effect could be produced by other forms of aural stimulation, provided that they were accompanied by 'appropriate suggestion'. Kenneth Bartlett, another research worker, called it simply 'hypnotism'. B. M. Schwaid warned that it might be hazardous because 'white noise' might damage the hearing of the patient. Gardner and Licklider fought back, claiming success in 90 per cent of 5,000 dental operations.

But in 1960, the Council on Dental Therapeutics voted to exclude an audio-analgesic device from its classification programme until more definite data was available. Sales of 'The Audio Analgesic' fell off.

In a report in *Oral Surgery* in 1964 (vol. 17, pp 319–24), Jack Rosenberg, Lecturer in Dental Psychology at the University of California, likened audio-analgesia to the 'confusion technique' sometimes used by hypnotists to get their patients into a trance,

> . . . in which contradictory and confusing statements are inserted into the induction 'patter', forcing the subject to concentrate all his effort and attention on an attempt to understand. This competing stimulus need not be white sound. It could just as easily be a recording of riveting or of horns honking, as long as it necessitates the attentive effort of the patient in order to hear the music through the interference. It is interesting to note that when audio-analgesia is produced in a good subject by a skilled operator, the white sound is seldom used.
>
> It is for these reasons that so many dentists have outstanding success when they try audio-analgesia for the first time, and are enthusiastic about the machine. Like children with a new toy, they impart enthusiasm and belief in the machine to their patients. The machine performs many of the functions that the hypnotist has to perform. Many patients are seeking magic remedies and often find them in the form of placebos. They now are offered a remedy for their fear of dental treatment. They are told how to act and what to expect. Then they are

presented with an overwhelming audio stimulus and 'an emergency white noise escape button'. The patient's head is filled with pleasant music, and we have the perfect setting for hypnosis. After the novelty of audio-analgesia wears off, the doctor who has the machine does not give the preliminary suggestions (mental set) as explicitly or as enthusiastically, and the phenomenon tends to be less effective.

In 1970, one of Dr Rosenberg's colleagues – Richard Weisbrod – summed up the state of audio-analgesia in these terms:

Since its introduction in 1959 by Gardner and Licklider, audio-analgesia has been the subject of much controversy. Part of this has been because of pronounced individual differences in its effects. In addition, some practitioners have experienced almost routine effectiveness while others have had unpredictable results.

R. K. Burt reported success in using audio-analgesia for relieving labor pains during childbirth. W. M. Moore, however, states that the results of his clinical trials of audioanalgesia in childbirth 'do not warrant continuation of the study in its present form'. Interestingly, he does note 'that three-quarters of the mothers (whether experimental or control) would like "sea-noise" again next time'. Audio-analgesia is apparently genuine, although its clinical effectiveness is not universally agreed upon. It is a complex and poorly understood psychophysiological phenomenon. The key to understanding it is closely tied to our knowledge of the underlying causes of pain perception. The audio-analgesic effect may provide important clues to the understanding of pain, and indeed, of the nervous system.

Audio-analgesia, once very popular, is not widely used today. The major objections to its clinical use seem to be (1) how it works is very poorly understood; (2) it is not effective for all patients; (3) its usefulness has not been demonstrated for all types of pain; and (4) its effect seems to be mostly 'psychological'.

Weisbrod adds: 'Audio-analgesia is not a panacea. While its limitations in use must be recognized, at the same time its advantages must not be ignored.'

★

Electrical methods

Dioscorides, a Greek surgeon operating at the time when Nero was Emperor of Rome, used to advocate the use of electric shocks from the torpedo fish as a relief from the pain of headache or neuralgia. He was, perhaps, the first to recognize the value of electricity as an anaesthetic.

In 1972, an instrument went on sale in Britain which consisted simply of two wires, a 22-volt battery, a meter and a pair of metal clips: one for connection to a dental drill, the other for attachment to the ear of a patient. Its function was to deliver a tingling sensation to the patient and so make him oblivious to pain. The equipment was designed in Russia, a country in which surgeons and dentists have made high claims for the effectiveness of the technique, and marketed in West Germany. Preliminary studies on a number of patients who volunteered to try it out, suggested that an effective level of anaesthesia could be induced if a steady current of between 45 and 60 milliamps was fed into the patient. In several drilling operations, which would normally have required the injection of a local anaesthetic, the patient felt no pain.

Discussing the machine in *Nature* (vol. 243, 22 June 1973), Dr P.P. Newman of Leeds University indicated that it had a sound physiological basis. He described an experiment with a frog:

> To demonstrate the method of anodal blocking, the frog's sciatic nerve was stimulated at its distal end by means of a square wave pulse generator, and the nerve action potentials, recorded from a proximal pair of electrodes, were displayed on an oscilloscope. The strength of the stimulus was arranged to produce a maximal response in order to excite all the individual fibres. When the output leads of the instrument were connected to a portion of the nerve between stimulating and recording electrodes, changes were induced by the flow of anodal current. As the strength of the current was increased, there was a progressive reduction in the amplitude of the action potentials with prolongation of conduction times until complete blockade was achieved. The depression was maintained during current flow and persisted for a few seconds after the current was switched off. Full recovery of the action potential was observed after about 10–15s. This procedure could be repeated many times without any obvious signs of fatigue in the nerves or changes in the form of the records.
>
> The potentials induced in a nerve membrane by an electrical stimulus are well known: the local state of polarization is disturbed and the membrane becomes freely permeable to ions. The depolarized region of the nerve-fibre initiates a local flow of current which extends into the adjacent resting membrane. This in turn becomes depolarized and a nerve-impulse is propagated along the fibre. The effect of an

applied anodal current is to oppose these changes either by restoring the polarized state or by producing hyperpolarization of the nerve membrane. The latter would account for the observed period of after-depression.

Dr Newman sums up:

Although the concept of anodal blocking of nerve-impulses has been evident for many years, its application to the clinical relief of pain is quite new. The apparent success of the method in dental anaesthesia is at least based on sound physiological principles, and it may become the method of choice for treatment of children and for very nervous patients, or for those with a high degree of sensitivity for pain. It is also possible, with suitable modifications, that the same principle could be applied to other regions of the body, for example in the treatment of fractures and emergency conditions that usually require the administration of a general anaesthetic.

Electro-anaesthesia is now being used with increasing success at the Necker Hospital in Paris on patients requiring urological surgery. It is intended for those patients for whom gas anaesthesia carries a high risk; for example, patients with renal, respiratory or cardiac insufficiency. Before the procedure, patients are given a tranquillizer followed by a local anaesthetic. Two positive connections are placed on the mastoids, and one negative on the forehead. A current is switched on and gradually raised to three milliamps in three minutes. Then waves of current (with a frequency of 120 kiloHertz) are sent through the head, in bursts of four thousandths of a second with eight thousandths of a second of 'rest' in between. When surgery is complete, the current is turned down to zero over a period of about one minute. The patient recovers consciousness, and remembers nothing of what has happened. So far, the Necker team have used the equipment on more than 150 patients for surgery lasting up to eight hours. Freedom from pain has been maintained for between two and twenty-four hours after the operation has been completed.

At the Centre for Pain Relief in Walton Hospital, Liverpool, surgeons have developed a technique for killing pain for two years or more by means of electric currents. It is called 'percutaneous cordotomy'. The electric current is used to kill nerves in the spine which carry pain from the affected part of the body to the brain. It has been used, so far, on more than 500 patients with otherwise incurable pain, and is said to have brought total relief to 85 per cent of them. Conditions treated have included 'phantom limb' pain, slipped discs, infection from the herpes virus (which can cause intense pain when it attacks nerves), and cancer.

In a report to *The Sunday Times*, Dr Oliver Gillie gave this description of a percutaneous cordotomy operation on a 48-year-old machine operator from the Ford Motor Company's Halewood plant:

Frank was completely conscious during the hour-long operation; this is necessary so that tests can be made to ensure that only pain-carrying nerve-fibres are destroyed. He was given a light pain-killing drug and a local anaesthetic, and then a hollow needle was stuck into the right side of his neck, passing between the first and second vertebrae, to touch the spinal cord.

Next, a wire was carefully positioned within the needle to touch exactly the part of the spinal cord which carried the pain messages. If the wire is placed two or three millimetres to one side, it would hit the motor nerve-fibres and cause paralysis down one side of the body. A millimetre or two in the other direction and the operation would achieve nothing. The target to be destroyed is a minute area of spinal cord about four millimetres square.

To help find this tiny target, a substance opaque to X-rays was injected into Frank's spinal canal. The needle and wire were placed in the correct position, using the X-ray screen. Then a test current was passed through the needle. Frank's right hand and foot twitched, showing that the needle was too far to one side and had to be moved a fraction. A second test then gave him pins and needles in his left hand, indicating that the wire was touching the pain-carrying fibres.

With the wire in the correct position, Frank was then asked to raise both his arms and his right leg. If the right arm or leg began to droop while the pain-carrying fibres were being destroyed, this would show that the destruction had gone far enough, and must be stopped. Electric diathermy current was switched on for a brief 2½-second burn. Immediately, Frank lost the feeling of pain coming from his left-hand side: a pin prick on that side now felt like the blunt prod of a finger. Two more brief burns, lasting eight seconds altogether, ensured that the pain-carrying fibres were totally destroyed. More tests showed that Frank's muscular control and strength of grip were completely unaffected by the operation.

A side-effect of the operation is loss of the sensation of hot and cold over the area where the feeling of pain has been lost. This is unavoidable because the same nerve-fibres carry both the sensation of pain and the sensation of hot and cold. After the operation, the patient must remember not to touch hot things with the affected side, or he could be burnt without feeling pain. But there is no loss of the sense of touch or any numbness over the area where the feeling of pain has been lost. The loss of pain lasts generally for two years or more, but the ability to feel pain will gradually return.

A 'do-it-yourself' electrical device for relieving certain common forms of acute and chronic pain was developed in the United States in the early 1970s. Called the 'Stimtech EPC Mini Stimulator', it weighed only thirty-four grammes (twelve ounces) and could be carried in a pocket or hooked on to a body-belt. Concealed wires led to electrodes which could be strapped or fixed with adhesive to a painful area, such as the back of the waist. A tingling current, obtained from the device's batteries, could be adjusted by the patient himself and left working for minutes or hours. According to its makers, it was able to 'block the transmission of pain messages through nerve-fibres to the brain by stimulating other fibres associated with them'.

'In one study,' the makers' report went on,

. . . electrical stimulation was successful in relieving 80 per cent of a group of patients incapacitated by chronic back trouble. In another, postoperative complications from abdominal surgery were reduced from one-in-three to one-in-sixteen, by allowing patients to clear their lungs by coughing, without the inhibition of pain.

Although no claims are made for curing the ailments which cause acute pain, electrical stimulation does often speed recovery, simply because concentrated physiotherapy is possible during pain-free periods.

Radiesthesia

Electrical apparatus of a more complex kind has been used for the diagnosis of disease and treatment of pain in the context of 'radiesthesia'. It first took the form of 'Abrams' Box'.

Radiesthesia is basically 'dowsing', or water-divining, applied to medical diagnosis. The radiesthetist believes that everything gives off radiations at different wavelengths, and that these are interpretable by him. To help discover the site and nature of disease or pain, he sometimes employs a pendulum. Just as a clairvoyant in a seance may use a wedding-ring suspended inside a glass to obtain tapped-out answers to questions, so the radiesthetist hopes his pendulum will swing and indicate the root of the trouble in the patient's body. Sometimes, the answer may come to him as a flash of inspiration: a single word emerging out of nothingness, either as a sound or a vision; sometimes, he may have to use a chart or a device like a ouija board, ringed with names of diseases and their remedies. Some radiesthetists begin treatment by picking up a succession of remedies in one hand, and 'feeling' from the movement of the pendulum in the other whether there is approval or disapproval. Others use their own hands for healing.

Albert Abrams was a neurologist practising in San Francisco. In 1902, he became interested in the use of radium in medical treatment and in the whole subject of radioactivity. He became convinced that radiations were universal to matter – a belief since accepted – and that since matter and energy were indistinguishable at the level of the atom, disease was more likely a disturbance of electrons than a disturbance of cells. He reasoned that it should be possible to build receiving equipment to detect the disturbance of radiation coming from a patient, and transmitting equipment to cure it.

He built a 'black box'. Then another, and another. Eventually he had a whole string of machines, which he hired out at a fee of 300 dollars a time, for diagnosing and treating disease. Not unnaturally, his fellow practitioners were scathing, even accusing him of fraudulent practice. But in 1924, a committee set up by the British Medical Association in London to investigate his claims came to the conclusion – after carefully supervised tests – that 'no more convincing exposition of the reality of this phenomenon could reasonably be desired'. The 'Abrams' box' did *something*, but how it worked they could not say. More research was called for.

Unfortunately, the funds for it were not forthcoming. Orthodox practitioners still poured scorn on the whole idea. However, variants of the 'box' were made – one by Dr Ruth Drown in America and another by George de la Warr in Oxford – and Dr T. B. B. Watson, President of the Medical Society for the Study of Radiesthesia, gives this description of how the diagnostic types work:

They consist of nine variable rheostats calibrated from 1 to 10, connected in series with a detector unit consisting of a thin sheet of rubber over a metal plate. They are not electrically powered. The patient may be directly linked to the instrument, or a blood-spot used. In the latter case, the patient may be any distance away, and it is believed that the information obtained from the instrument refers to the state of the patient at the time of the examination. A vibration-rate has been allotted to each organ and tissue in health and disease, as well as to parasites, bacteria, viruses, chemicals, hormones, vitamins, and so on. These rates are represented by numbers which, however, bear no relation to any known physical vibration-rate.

In making a diagnosis, organ-rates are set up in turn on the dials. To determine the energy output of any organ, the rubber pad is stroked with the finger while the ninth dial is rotated from 10 to 1. At the number representing the energy of the organ, the rubber becomes sticky to the finger. To discover the nature of the pathological condition of the organ, disease-rates are set up on the dials. In this way, it is claimed that a complete picture of the state of the mind and the body of the patient may be determined. As in map-dowsing and diagnosis by pendulum, anatomical diagrams may be used. A pointer connected to the instrument is moved over the diagram while the detector-pad is being operated, and the precise site of the lesion detected. In this instrument also, the mind of the operator plays a dominant part. At each item under investigation the operator has to say to himself, 'Has this patient got so-and-so?' Some consider that this instrument is a guide to the mind and that the information it gives is found by a subjective method akin to psychometry.

A treatment 'box' was also developed by Ruth Drown which was said to 'place the individual in series with the instrument and use his own energy as a means of treatment, even as Nature does when a cut finger is to be healed'. Claims were made that it could alleviate pain in rheumatism.

In 1960, a court-case was brought in Britain against George de la Warr, alleging that his 'box' was a fraud. How could something whose leads were connected to magnets, dials and rheostats – but not to any source of power, nor even to the patient – possibly work? The operator who brought the action said that, according to indications given by the 'box', the sex of her patients 'appeared to change from day to day'. The judge did not rule on whether or not the 'box' worked; but he did say that he was convinced that George de la Warr honestly believed in his device and his methods, and was not, therefore, guilty of fraud.

Today, a few diagnostic and treatment 'boxes' are still in use; in

1962, *The Observer*'s racing correspondent described how one had been used to diagnose a displaced lumbar vertebra in a racehorse called Scotch Delinquent (by examining a few hairs from its tail), and how a 'treatment' had been broadcast from the 'box' to the racehorse. But generally speaking, interest in radiesthesia has focused more on its manipulative aspects, and on its relationships with homeopathy, than on its electronic powers – if, that is, they exist.

Homeopathy

Christian Friedrich Samuel Hahnemann was born at Meissen, Saxony, in 1755. He studied medicine at Leipzig and Vienna, qualified as a physician, and returned to Leipzig to practice in 1789. But he was sickened by what he regarded as the 'blunderbuss' approach and brutality of many of his fellow physicians, and soon gave up his practice in favour of pharmacological research.

A year later, while translating *Materia Medica* – the great compendium of herbal remedies drawn up by W. Cullen – he was struck by the fact that the symptoms produced by quinine in the human body were the same as those of the sick state it was supposed to cure; or, as Sir John Weir put it later, 'while diligently seeking the light, it suddenly flamed before his eyes . . . there could be no doubt about it: quinine both caused and cured ague.'

Hahnemann reasserted the truth of an ancient doctrine, *similia similibus curantur*: 'like likes to be treated by like'. He suggested that the quinine acted by triggering an 'antagonistic fever' which counteracted the ague. He labelled his theory 'homeopathy', after the Greek *homoios* (meaning 'like') and *pathos* (meaning 'suffering').

Over the next four years, he propounded a fuller doctrine based upon 'simples' – single substances extracted from natural sources such as herbs or minerals – which he tried in ever-decreasing doses and found to be even more potent in small amounts than in large. These 'micro-doses' appeared to stimulate the body's own defences. This principle became Rule 2 of homeopathy.

Rule 3 was, 'Treat the patient rather than the disease.' This was arrived at by the logic that if the patient's own defences were to be strengthened, his individuality had to be understood – his background, constitution and temperament – because each patient was different.

Hahnemann's three principles have remained to this day. He himself was hounded, but he acquired disciples. One of these was Frederick Foster Harvey Quin, an Englishman who studied under Hahnemann and returned to become the first homeopathic practitioner in Britain. He had a difficult time of it, too. 'I stood alone in England,' he wrote later, 'isolated from all my medical brethren, listened to with suspicion, looked upon with coolness by my early professional friends, exposed constantly to the shafts of ridicule, to illiberal representation and to the severest and most bitter censure, with no one to consult or share responsibility.' But he persevered, and soon he was joined by others.

The first homeopathic hospital was set up in Golden Square, London in 1850. Today there are about 250 homeopathic practitioners in Britain – slightly fewer than in Quin's time – but the homeopath's *Materia medica* contains some 2,000 therapeutic substances, many of them useful in the alleviation of pain. For headaches there are at least ten, including belladonna, aconite, Spigelia and the kali salts.

Here are some typical case reports from presently-practising homeopaths:

Case 1. 'A boy of ten came complaining of shooting-pain around the left eye followed by sickness and occurring at monthly intervals. He was chilly, highly strung and easily worried. He was friendly but obstinate, rather untidy and weepy. More on the local than the general symptoms, I prescribed Spigelia 30, expecting that he might require a more general constitutional remedy to follow. However, two months later he had only had two short attacks without sickness, and had been able to go to school on each occasion. Spigelia was repeated twice and he was free of all headache for four months between.'

Case 2. 'A housewife, aged thirty-four, with rheumatoid arthritis for nine years. She had received treatment at the Charterhouse Clinic, but had steadily deteriorated. She received Medorrhinum CM, one dose, followed by Rhus. tox. 1M and CM. She began to improve within a month, and eighteen months later was still improving. *Comment:* the degree of her disability and the quality of her improvement are not specified, but it is clear that the "turn of the tide" from deterioration to improvement occurred soon after taking the high potencies.'

Case 3. 'A male clerk, aged fifty-eight, had sciatica for four years. Phytolacca IM, three doses, produced a dramatic improvement within ten days. One year later the pain recurred, and he took three more doses, which were followed by complete remission. Follow-up for four years; no more pain. *Comment:* the cause of the sciatica was not proved by radiography, he was not referred to hospital, but was previously treated by analgesics.'

Case 4. 'A receptionist, aged eighteen, strained a knee for the third time in one year. Ruta 10M, three doses at twelve-hour intervals, produced a rapid improvement which surprised the patient, who compared it with the slow improvement on the two former occasions. Follow-up for four weeks; no further trouble. *Comment:* Ruta is valuable for injuries to ligaments.'

And so forth. One of the prime objections of orthodox practitioners to homeopathy is that it is slow to produce results: 'micro-doses' do not usually produce spectacular effects, and improvement takes time. However, there exist thousands of patients eager to testify to its efficacy, who are less fearful of homeopathic treatments than of those based on allopathy: treatments which produce phenomena *unlike* those of the disease they are treating.

It is, like so many things in medicine, a matter of individual choice.

Old Wives' Tales

'If you get a touch of lumbago,' my grandmother used to declare, 'carry a potato in your pocket, and it will soon go away.'

'Why?' I asked.

'Well, it soaks up the moisture in the air which makes lumbago *feel* worse,' she would explain. And there, in my own family, was a classic example of an Old Wives' Tale.

Many Old Wives' Tales for relieving pain are myths, pure and simple. But some contain a grain of truth. For instance, in the case of rheumatic-type pain, damp weather conducts away more body-heat than usual, with the result that the victim often *feels* pain more in damp conditions. The potato in the pocket is, presumably, supposed to absorb some of this dampness.

'If you get cramp in the night, go to bed with a bundle of corks,' is another common Old Wives' Tale. Indeed, in 1973 it provoked considerable correspondence in the journals of the Women's Institute; some writers favoured putting the feet on to a cork mat beside the bed. I have tried both 'cures'. Neither worked in my case, although the slight softness and warmth of the cork mat did induce a minor relaxation of the calf muscles, and brought temporary relief, therefore, from the cramp. However, it soon returned.

Probably the most common Old Wives' analgesic is copper. Every week, newspaper advertisements for expensive copper bangles lure victims of arthritis, rheumatism or similarly painful disorders to part with their money in the hope of finding relief. Homeopaths see nothing surprising in this.

'It is only in the homeopathic school of medical therapeutics that copper is used with any demonstrable success and surety of purpose,' writes Dr Anthony Shupis in the *Journal of the American Institute of Homeopathy* (Sept.-Oct. 1965).

> With its similars – camphor and *veratrum album* – it must be considered in the following states: acute myocardial infarction, angina pectoris, cholera, infectious diarrhoea of the newborn, asthma, cramps, croup, hysteria, neuralgias, influenza and whooping cough. . . . It has worked wonders in many cases of dysmenorrhea. . . . Cramps in the legs respond more completely to it than to any other single remedy I am aware of.

According to homeopaths like Dr Shupis, the copper works because the conditions he mentions all have symptoms similar to those which can be produced by copper poisoning; the copper, therefore, acts as an antagonist when applied in minute doses. Dr Shupis also throws some light on the habit of wearing copper next to the skin:

> There is a practice, growing in the United States, of the wearing of copper chains. Its origin is obscure. This practice has been mentioned in relation to cholera and cholera countries, but in the United States, where cholera is no longer present, the wearing of copper chains is supposed to be helpful to rheumatism and arthritis sufferers. It came to the attention of the Somers Brass Co., rollers of thin-sheet metals, through one of their salesmen. It seems that an acquaintance of this salesman bought a set of copper chains, wrapped in a fancy box, for about seven or eight dollars. Knowing, from business experience, that a goodly percentage of these chains were and are produced by The Bead Chain Manufacturing Co. of Bridgeport, Connecticut, for use as pull-chains for light-bulbs, key rings, etc., Somers Brass ordered some and gave them *gratis* to their customers, or whoever might request them. They made no claims but in many cases received gratifying letters for help received by these chains. They have since discontinued the practice. For anyone of the homeopathic persuasion, there is no doubt that in some instances, if the symptoms of the wearer match those of copper – particularly with the crampy element that appears in the older people – it can easily be seen how this crude form of unconscious homeopathy can be helpful.

9

A World without Pain?

We should, perhaps, be grateful for pain. It is Nature's early-warning system, telling us that something is wrong. Ignore it, if it persists, and the consequences may be devastating: pleurisy perhaps, cystitis, a fractured bone, perforated ulcer or even a 'coronary'. Ignore the pin-pricking pain of a splinter, and sepsis may follow; ignore a headache after a rugby tackle, and permanent brain damage may result.

The most common pain is the one indicating the need to urinate: who would wish to be without *that* warning pain?

Consider, too, what may happen when pain is incautiously relieved. Injection of a steroid into an arthritic joint can relieve pain dramatically. But the result may be that the joint is thereafter used by the patient in such a way that it deteriorates faster. For this reason, a doctor will rarely, if ever, give a pain-killer until he is sure of his diagnosis, for fear of distorting or masking some vital sign which may enable him to pin-point the site of the damage, or the underlying cause in the body.

It would be of no benefit to anyone if there were a world without pain. What we must seek to conquer is *useless* pain, or unnecessarily intense pain: the pain of irreversible disease; agonizing causalgia following damage to a nerve; the pains of menstruation, childbirth, migraine and suchlike.

What are the prospects?

Fresh discoveries about the mechanism of pain, the action of certain natural substances in the body, and the development of new techniques for treating chronic pain, promise a new measure of relief on a wider scale than hitherto. A whole new medical speciality is developing – dolorology. Using treatment ranging from massive surgery to transcendental meditation, the dolorologists are attacking chronic pain from many quarters. 'It is one of the most dramatic things happening in medicine', was how Dr Donlin Long, director of the Johns Hopkins Pain Treatment Centre described it when I spoke to him.

Until recently, the average chronic-pain patient in America suffered for seven years, underwent three to five major operations and spent between $50,000 and $100,000 on doctors' bills. Things were a little better in Britain but not much. In between operations, countless drugs were swallowed – often with the result that the pain-sufferer became a drug addict. But new approaches to the conquest of pain are now being made.

Ideally, the answer to the problem of persistent pain will be found in the fields of pharmacology and medical chemistry. The search for the perfect analgesic continues ceaselessly (the perfect analgesic being a drug with only one specific action – the relief of pain). Such a drug should not cause vomiting, should not affect the circulation or depress the respiration. It should be free of any tendency to bring about tolerance and not be habit-forming. There are signs that such a substance may be attainable.

In 1973, Dr Solomon Snyder of the Johns Hopkins School of Medicine in Baltimore, and Candice Pert of the US National Institute of Mental Health, discovered during the course of basic research on drug addiction that there are clusters of cells in certain parts of the brain which attract narcotics. They reasoned that Nature would not put these 'opiate receptors' into the brain just to accumulate *man-made* narcotics: their function was probably to respond to *natural* opiate-like substances produced in the body – perhaps for the very purpose of controlling pain.

Two years later, workers in the Unit for Research on Addictive Drugs at Aberdeen University, who were collaborating with a research team at Reckitt & Colman, isolated a substance from the brains of pigs which appeared to act like morphine and was attracted by the 'opiate receptors' in the brain just like the man–made narcotics. They named it enkephalin ('in the head') and nicknamed it 'the brain's own opiate'.

It was a major discovery. Dr Roger Lewin, writing in *New Scientist* (1 January 1976), commented:

> With the structure of enkephalin now at hand, we are now poised for an exciting breakthrough in the complete understanding of opiate analgesia, addiction and tolerance. Probably the most intriguing aspect of all this is the inescapable implication that there exists in the brain an unexpected 'chemical transmitter system' – a system which may have something to do with dampening pain, but almost certainly has more general effects also.

A race against time began. Other researchers, in Sweden and the USA, reported finding a similar substance in the brains of mice, rats and rabbits. Having isolated the substance, the British team – led by Dr John Hughes and Professor H. W. Kosterlitz at Aberdeen – set about trying to purify it. Most of the molecule's structure was worked out by one of their colleagues at Aberdeen, Linda Fothergil. But the work was advanced considerably by a peptide chemist with Reckitt & Colman, Barry Morgan, who helped to show that enkephalin was, in fact, a conventional peptide made up from a sequence of amino acids. But when it came to analysing that sequence, Morgan was as puzzled as the rest of them.

At this point, the research story became rather extraordinary.

The team turned for help to a spectroscopist, Howard Morris of Imperial College, London, who was able to show that *two* peptides were present – not one. Synthesis of all the materials was then achieved, and the man-made version was found to correspond exactly with natural enkephalin. Each contained five amino acids, with one being present in quantities three times greater than the others. But *where* did enkephalin come from in the body, and *how* did it act?

A curious quirk of Fate then occurred. Still pondering on the exact nature of the substance, Howard Morris attended a lecture at Imperial College given by a visiting speaker, Derek Smythe of the National Institute for Medical Research. Smythe's subject was a protein called Beta-lipotropin, and he showed a sequence of slides indicating its chemical structure.

Suddenly, to his amazement, Morris recognized the outlines of enkephalin embedded in the molecular diagrams showing the structure of Beta-lipotropin. There, quite clearly, was the peptide, in position – part of the routine output of the pituitary gland. Dr Roger Lewin takes up the technical explanation:

> The first four out of the five amino acids had not been difficult to settle: they are tyrosine-glycine-glycine-phenylalanine. It was the fifth that proved tricky. Standard analyses had shown variable amounts of methionine and leucine. The reason now is clear: one peptide has methionine at the end (met-enkephalin), and the other has leucine (leu-enkephalin); the ratio between the two peptides (in the pig) is about 3:1 respectively. . . .

Morris noticed that embedded in the β-lipotropin sequence (residues 61 to 65) was enkephalin, the methionine variety.

Dr Lewin goes on:

This is all the more intriguing because residues 41 to 58 of β-lipotropin are identical with β-melanocyte stimulating hormone (β-MSH). β-lipotropin appears to be the natural parent of β-MSH which is formed when the excess amino acids are snipped off by protease enzymes. Could β-lipotropin also be the parent of met-enkephalin? This is certainly a possibility. But then there is the problem of the origin of leu-enkephalin. Might there be a yet to be discovered β-lipotropin with a leucine residue at position 65? Again, this is possible, but Smythe says he is sceptical.

The discovery of yet another behaviourally active peptide manufactured in the pituitary gland makes the list of such molecules even longer, and it adds another twist to the structurally incestuous relationships apparent between them.

Dr Lewin continues:

Analgesia is, of course, what interests the pharmaceutical companies, because they would like to produce a powerful pain-killer which is not addictive, a major drawback of the standard opiates. Analogues of enkephalin, still at a very experimental stage, are said to be promising as possible analgesics; shortening the molecule by just one amino acid, however, has disastrous results on the biological potency, reducing it to about 1 per cent.

Another exciting research thrust just beginning at Aberdeen is determining the exact intracellular location of enkephalin. Answers from this will settle the question of whether enkephalin is a neurotransmitter itself, or whether it works by modifying the activity of others. And from this there will be important leads on the function of enkephalin. New brain chemicals are not *so* rare these days, but enkephalin is the most intriguing found recently.

The Endorphins

Since then, researchers in different parts of the world have found no less than seven enkephalin-like compounds in the brain or bloodstream. Unfortunately, experiments have shown that they are almost as addictive as morphine – ruling out the possibility, for the present, of the 'perfect' pain-killer. But research into 'the endorphins', as the whole group of substances is now known, has thrown new light on our understanding of the mechanism of pain, and of other brain functions as well. Enkephalins turn out to be located in precisely those areas of the brain where Professors Melzack and Wall – the 'gate theorists' – place their 'central biasing mechanism' (the spring which can close the 'gate' from within the brain if it does not want to admit pain-signals).

At a meeting of the American Society of Neuroscience at Anaheim, California, in November 1977, Dr Solomon Snyder reported that he had been able to map specific nerve pathways in the brain where the substances act. One such pathway was in the limbic system – the region thought to be involved in emotional behaviour. 'It could well be', added Dr Snyder, 'the pathway that has to do with the mechanism of euphoria.'

Other researchers speculated that *lack* of enkephalins – or a paucity of 'opiate receptors' – may explain why some people are hypersensitive to pain. 'We are starting to understand, also,' said Dr Snyder, 'how the brain regulates mood. It is quite conceivable that any number of mental disease states could be related to abnormalities in the enkephalins.'

While work on the endorphins goes on apace, a group of scientists in Sweden – Thomas Hökfelt and his colleagues at the Karolinska Institute, Stockholm – have thrown fresh light on a substance, originally discovered in the 1930s by the eminent neuro-pharmacologist Von Euler, known as 'Substance P'.

Substance P

Substance P, according to the Swedish research, may be the messenger which carries pain-signals along nerves through the body to the brain. Hökfelt and his team have not only found traces of Substance P in the brains of cats and rats but also in the sensory nerves going into their spinal cords; it is *not* present, however, in the motor nerves (controlling movement) leaving the spinal cord. Could it be, they wonder, that Substance P is a transmitter for sensory information?

The Swedish team used fluorescent dyes to light up the nerve-endings which contained Substance P. They traced the fluorescence not only to cells in the brain but also to sensory cells in the peripheral nervous system; and not only to the main body of each cell but to the tiny fibres (known as C-fibres) which extend out to the sense-organs in the skin. These fibres are believed to transmit information about pressure, temperature and pain.

It would seem that Substance P transmits pain information all the way from the source of the pain to the decoding centre in the brain. But, as the *New Scientist* said in an annotation in December 1975:

Although Hökfelt has produced a tentative answer to some of the questions surrounding Substance P, many more remain to be answered. One very basic one is whether, in fact, Substance P is itself a neurotransmitter; or whether it modulates in some way the action of other neurotransmitters. Another is whether there is just one Substance P or a family of closely related substances. . . . The fluorescent antibody turned up in all sorts of areas of the brain, not only those which normally accept sensory messages. What is it doing there? Only more research will tell.

While neurologists and neuro-pharmacologists tackle these new questions in the puzzle that is pain, others are continuing the search for more effective treatments. Unfortunately, the assessment of 'effectiveness' is not easy.

A variety of animal tests are used to assess a new analgesic. In man, experimental pains can be produced by pricking, pressure or heat; the drug is then given to the volunteer and his reactions noted. But all such tests depend upon personal observations or testimony, which makes objective evaluation of the pain-killer almost impossible. What is needed is a really accurate 'pain thermometer', something that will enable a doctor to say, 'Mrs Bloggs is in severe pain; she has 18 degrees of pain, or 26 ounces or 45 centimetres.'

Harold Wolff, the neurologist, tried hard to develop such an instrument many years ago. He proved that humans can distinguish between twenty-two levels of pain, ranging from 'threshold' (the level at which it is first felt) to 'ceiling' (the point at which increased stimulation produces no additional pain). He called each pair of steps in the pain ladder a 'dol'. But his 'dolorimeter' is an inexact instrument. Nobody really knows whether clinical pain – the pain of arthritis, a heart attack, surgery, or whatever suffering a human being has in daily life – is the same as the pain which the investigator produces experimentally on his human subjects in the research laboratory.

The difference between the forms of pain is considerable where the sufferer's psychological reaction is concerned, for a sudden pain whose meaning is unknown, even in the course of the ordinary day's routine, will produce a distinct reaction: fear and anxiety usually accompany most of our hurts until we feel certain no damage has been done. Fear and anxiety may, of course, be allowed by giving a tranquillizing agent in conjunction with a pain-killer, and improved combinations of drugs will undoubtedly be devised in the future, so that *every* patient – even if not completely spared pain – will at least be able to say, 'Doctor, I still feel the pain, but it doesn't *bother* me so much.'

Pain Clinics

Overcoming fear and anxiety is also one of the chief rationales for Pain Clinics, special units dedicated to the relief of pain, some fifty of which have been set up in Britain and America so far. Those who work in them believe that many more should be set up in future. Dr Cicely Saunders, who runs such a clinic in south-east London with the aid of a team of nuns, comments:

> Most important, perhaps, is *listening*: listening in order to analyse the patient's situation, and to attend as a person ready to be aware not only of the nature of the pain on the physical level, but also of its implication for this individual with his own culture and background, past experience and present anxieties. Talking about pain or other symptoms may be a way out of talking about more serious concerns, but it can also be a way in, or a way of conveying reassurance at a much deeper level.
>
> Communication without words, or at least with indirect ones, is often the most important communication that takes place, and it is such talk that gives the opportunity for recognizing the moment when the real question is not: 'What do you tell your patients?' but rather: 'What do you let your patients tell you?' This means attention not only to details of the story and to the facts of the physical part of the pain but also to all the various symptoms that may accompany it, and to their treatment. Sometimes patients will complain bitterly of a minor trouble, which may distract the attention of the doctor (and their own) from more major concerns that are too threatening to look at. So often it *is* the apparently small thing that is the problem. So much 'pain' can be relieved by symptomatic treatment, by nursing measures, control of intercurrent infections, attention to diet, and so on.

Her experience is borne out by specialists at King's College Hospital, London:

> In many cases, the patients are referred to the clinic with long histories of persistent, intractable pain. They appear to find great relief in having the opportunity to discuss their own particular case-history at great length with the doctor; and it has been found that the chance to have a lengthy, sympathetic discussion is of great therapeutic value in itself, even if it only be psychological.

Radical Treatments

Types of intractable pain dealt with in such Pain Clinics are diverse, ranging from cancer, inoperable heart disease and orthopaedic pain to vascular problems, neuralgia, and rare and strange conditions. Apart from relieving pain, the Clinics frequently enable hospital in-patients to be released earlier than usual, thereby freeing desperately-needed beds.

A comprehensive review of the more radical procedures used by the Pain Clinics was given at a symposium, 'Pain and Pain Relief', held at the Wembley Conference Centre on 20 October 1977 under the auspices of Merck, Sharp and Dohme. One of the speakers, Dr Samson Lipton, Director of the Centre for Pain Relief at Walton Hospital, Liverpool, described two different surgical approaches – one for inoperable diseases such as cancer, and the other for treating non-malignant conditions.

'In a way,' he told the conference,

> . . . it is much easier to treat cancer pain than any other type of pain (because the chances are that the patient will not live long enough for the body to regenerate pain-sensitivity after the treatment has been given). The easiest method is to destroy the part of the central nervous system which carries the pain. We use a number of techniques – all of which hinge on the use of the X-ray Image Intensifier – but the three main ones are antero-lateral cordotomy, pituitary destruction by alcohol, and subarachnoid phenol blocking.

Dr Lipton went on: 'Antero-lateral cordotomy is useful for cancer pain which is unilateral and below shoulder-level – in the arm, the body or the leg – and it is effective in about 90 per cent of patients. You knock out the antero-lateral nerve, and the patient becomes absolutely free of pain. I personally have done about 700 of these operations and they take between 45 and 60 minutes – they work, they really do.'

For disseminated cancer pain, he continued, pituitary destruction was the preferred method, although it was only successful in about 70 per cent of cases.

> You put a longish needle through the spaces of the nose, through the sphenoid sinus and into the pituitary fossa, and you inject about one millilitre of alcohol into it. This destroys the pituitary gland to a large extent, and can be repeated. It relieves pain completely in 40 per cent of patients, and partially in 30 per cent.

The subarachnoid phenol blocks – our third method – have been known for a long time, but they are used today in a rather different fashion to the way they were originally used, with far fewer side-effects. The trouble is, they don't last very long.

Injections of phenol and glycerin, as a way of *chemically* interrupting the pathway of pain, were first tried out in 1953. The mixture is injected into the subarachnoid space, a narrow channel which contains the cerebro-spinal fluid. Relief experienced by patients continues for up to fifteen months, but the injections are not easy to perform and bladder complications sometimes follow. A variation of the technique is to flush the cerebro-spinal fluid with ice-cold saline. This method has practically no side-effects, but relief only lasts from one to five months, although the procedure can be repeated.

Nerve-blocking may be done in several ways: by injecting phenol and glycerine, or an ice-cold saline solution, into the fluid in the spinal column; by passing an electric current through a wire positioned at the top of the spine; or by stimulating particular nerve-fibres in the spinal cord with radio signals.

Describing the last procedure in detail (*Nursing Times*, 24 August 1973), Dr John Lloyd of Abingdon Hospital, Berkshire – where Britain's very first Pain Clinic was established – claimed 'a high degree of success' with it.

It involves the implantation of a radio-frequency electrode in the subarachnoid space overlying the posterior columns of the spinal cord. Stimuli are provided by a radio-frequency transmitter which may be carried in the patient's pocket, and a succession of sensory stimuli are delivered to the posterior columns in the cord. This has the effect of preventing the discharge from the small-diameter fibres which tend to carry pain and, in many patients who have had intractable pain, the use of this stimulator has given them complete pain relief for as long as the stimulation lasts. It is in essence extremely similar to a cardiac pacemaker, but instead of stimulating the heart it is stimulating nerve-tissue.

The Case of the Vietnam Veteran

Such portable stimulators are also widely used in America. One patient delighted with his is Joe Lyttle, whose ordeal began in Vietnam in 1968 when enemy gunfire brought down his helicopter. A bullet hit him in the back, paralysing him from the waist down.

'What was worse', he recalls now, 'was the pain. It would start with the feeling you have when your legs have been asleep and then start to wake up. Then I would get this real sharp, burning sensation – like my legs were being stripped of flesh and the wind was blowing hard on them.'

For two months, he was given heavy doses of narcotics. But doctors at the veterans hospital to which he was admitted, refused to believe he could be in pain because of the paralysis: 'They told me that I was numb from the waist down and that it was impossible for my legs to hurt.' For the next five years, he went from doctor to doctor in search of relief. A psychiatrist told him the pain was psychological – due to the fact that he was unwilling to accept being paralysed. A chiropractor was able to give some relief with massage. Then a surgeon attempted nerve-block by injecting first Novocaine, then alcohol. But the operation had to be halted: 'The Novocaine felt like it had set me on fire,' recalls Lyttle.

Finally, he went to a Pain Clinic. He saw Dr C. Norman Shealy of La Crosse, Wisconsin, who implanted tiny wires in the dorsal column of his spinal cord, attached to an electronic receiver implanted under the skin of his back. He was issued with a small control-unit which could be slipped into his shirt pocket, and which supplied current to the implanted stimulator.

Lyttle, now nearing forty and living with his wife and daughter in Fisherville, Virginia, has been diagnosed as suffering from 'paraplegic-pain syndrome' – a rare type of affliction similar to the 'phantom limb' pain felt by some amputees. He still suffers occasional bouts of pain 'like a red-hot coal in my hip-joint'. But he has been able to hold down a job as a recreational supervisor at a rehabilitation centre – despite being in a wheelchair – and goes hunting. The key to his freedom is the stimulator which produces, every waking moment of the day, a vibration through the lower part of his body and dulls the pain.

Other Vibrations

Vibrations of a rather different kind are now being tried for the relief of less acute but equally chronic pains. Technically, they are known as 'cycloid low-frequency vibration therapy', or 'cyclomassage' for short.

The equipment consists of a mains-powered motor which creates low-frequency vibrations. It can be secreted inside a cushion or pad, or installed as part of the bed, or handled as a 'stroker' and passed by hand over affected parts of the body. The latest version, described as 'perfect for the hardworking businessman', can be incorporated in a chair.

'Cyclomassage', at the time of writing, is in use in some fifty British hospitals and is the subject of evaluation by (among others) the Medical Research Council, Royal College of Surgeons and Birmingham Medical School. One early report on its use – from the Robert B. Bingham Hospital in Boston, Massachusetts – spoke of its value in the treatment of rheumatoid arthritis. Twenty-six patients tried it and it proved to be 'simple, safe and effective'. The report added: 'Of practical importance, from the patients' viewpoint, is the observation that the repeated daily use of this equipment by the patient resulted in an increase in the activities of daily living which was of great importance to the patient.'

Another early assessment – made at a hospital in North-East England – reported benefit from cyclomassage to sufferers from low-back pain. 'There was little to choose between it and diathermy,' it concluded. Such vibrators probably achieve their effect by distraction: 'The patient may know the pain is there but, by focusing attention on something else, you can filter out the hurt,' was how one practitioner put it. But 'distracting' methods are virtually useless in the face of severe, intractable pain. Probably the fastest-growing method favoured by the Pain Clinics is percutaneous electrical cordotomy which, as indicated earlier, calls for a wire to be positioned carefully in the spinal column to knock out specific nerve-fibres.

First, a needle is inserted into the spino-thalamic tract under guidance from an X-ray monitor. A fine wire is then fed through the needle, and an electric current sent down it. The passage of the current tends to be painful but patients are mentally prepared to withstand it, and if the electrical method is unsuccessful open cordotomy (physical cutting of the nerve-fibre) can be performed later.

Drastic surgery is only used as a last resort. As Mr R. D. Illingworth of the Central Middlesex Hospital pointed out in 1973 (*British Journal of Hospital Medicine*, May 1973):

> Surgical treatment of pain falls into two distinct groups. First, there are operations for specific painful conditions, particularly trigeminal neuralgia, and secondly, operations to treat pain arising as one of the symptoms in conditions such as malignant disease. . . . When considering the possibility of an operation in a patient with pain due to some benign condition, one should remember that pain is not necessarily an abnormal sensation. To feel pain may be essential for survival, and to abolish the sensation of pain from a part of the body is in a way a mutilating operation. After a few years, there is a tendency for pain to return, which is another reason to hesitate before

performing cordotomy or posterior rhizotomy on a patient whose disease is not likely to be fatal. Sometimes a patient with pain due to a benign cause has a series of operations, each one of which leaves the patient in a worse state than before. It is better not to embark on this course, which can cause much distress to both patient and doctor.

One of the 'specific painful conditions' to which Mr Illingworth referred – trigeminal neuralgia – involves cutting a nerve or nerves in the face. One patient who has benefited from such surgery is Evelyn Moreland, a 58-year-old housewife in Pittsburgh, Pennsylvania, who first felt the pain in her face twenty-three years ago when she wiped her hand over her forehead.

One morning, she woke to feel throbbing, surging pain over the whole of the left side of her face: 'You couldn't believe how bad it was, it just knocked me out.'

Over the next twenty years, Mrs Moreland's condition – diagnosed as *tic douloureux* – became progressively worse. She would feel sharp pains about the face, followed by ten or fifteen minutes of exhaustion. 'The pain was so bad', she recalls, 'that I wanted to tear my hair out. There were many times when I couldn't eat, brush my teeth or touch my face. A puff of wind would set it off.' She tried pain-killing drugs and anti-convulsants. But they made her tired and weak. Eventually she agreed to surgery. An operation was performed at the Presbyterian Hospital, Pittsburgh, in which pressure on the offending nerve was relieved – and the neuralgia disappeared.

But the memory lingers on. 'I still hesitate before leaving the house on a windy day,' admits Mrs Moreland, 'and when I kiss people I still turn my right cheek to them – so that they won't touch my left.'

New operations for the relief of pain are still tried experimentally but they tend to be minor rather than major. One radical procedure – leucotomy (in which nerves leading to the brain itself are severed) – has recently fallen from favour.

Leucotomy tends to affect the patient's perception of pain rather than his actual reactions to it. A survey carried out in 1958 first questioned its value (Elithorn and others, *Journal of Neurology, Neurosurgery and Psychiatry*, vol. 21, p. 249) by reporting that only 35 per cent of patients who had undergone the operation, and 38 per cent of their relatives, felt that the surgery had been worthwhile. Since then, marked personality-changes have been noted in leucotomized patients. Nevertheless, less drastic surgical procedures find widespread support amongst patients attending pain clinics today. Dr John Lloyd of Abingdon reports:

> Most of our patients prefer to have some form of nerve-block performed to control their pain, so that they can forget about it and go back home to lead as normal a life as possible. They maintain that if they are given drugs, they are unable to forget the pain because if they forgot to take the tablets the pain would return. Many patients who have had successful nerve-blocks have been pain-free, working, and leading a relatively normal life for as long as twelve months.

The whole future of Pain Clinics in Britain has recently been studied by the British Pain Society. It concluded that every District Hospital – serving, perhaps, 250,000 people – should have a specialist on its staff offering two or three sessions per week for dealing with chronic pain cases. Furthermore, regional or teaching hospitals should have at least one clinician (preferably two) with supporting staff, devoted to the problems of pain. Such changes in the allocation of hospital services could be introduced almost over-night – but are unlikely to be, because of conservatism and a short-age of National Health Service funds. But the benefits are now plainly apparent.

In the meantime, one may reasonably expect two quite different advances to be made towards the conquest of pain: one is in the development of new analgesic 'delivery systems', the other in the use of mental 'conditioning' of patients.

New methods are under investigation by the pharmaceutical industry for positioning 'depots' of analgesic in or on the body, so that only a controlled amount of drug is released over a period of hours or days. With a condition such as arthritis of the knee, a depot of aspirin may be placed in the synovial fluid of the knee itself, so that a tiny quantity would seep slowly and combat the pain without passing through the patient's stomach. Such a technique, if it can be perfected, would completely overcome the problem of gastric irritation.

'Strap-on' drugs are also the subject of present-day research. The substance is held against the skin – for example, just behind the ear – so that it seeps through into the bloodstream over a period of days, a method of getting the maximum benefit out of some analgesics.

But perhaps the most immediate step which could be taken towards the further conquest of pain is in the field of mental 'condi-tioning'. We all know how human response to pain varies according to mental attitude: a bruise collected in the course of a game, or while dealing with some emergency, may not be noticed, whereas quite minor pains may be magnified by dwelling on them.

A fresh and most striking psychiatric approach to the relief of pain is through hypnosis. What the hypnotist teaches his patient is how to handle pain so that it cannot overwhelm him. 'The patient learns to superimpose a feeling of numbness over the pain area and to filter the hurt out of it,' one medical hypnotist told me. 'He does this by focusing his awareness on something else, as if he were absorbed in some task. It's like trying to take your mind off a broken leg by biting your finger.'

With hypnosis, many victims of incurable cancer have had their morphine dosage reduced by two-thirds, or even eliminated. Although only about 20 per cent of patients go into a deep trance, a further 60 per cent are said to succumb sufficiently to have their perception of pain reduced.

The ability of mind to triumph over matter is well illustrated by a study of 97 patients at the Massachusetts General Hospital, who were divided, on the eve of undergoing abdominal surgery, into two groups: one group was told what pain to expect after the operation (the pain of muscle spasm under the incision), and how to reduce it by relaxing the muscles; the other was told nothing. Afterwards, with nurses and doctors ignorant as to which patient was in which group, it was found that those who had been mentally 'conditioned' requested only half as much analgesic as the others. Furthermore, they were able to go home an average of 2.7 days earlier. Commenting on these findings, Dr Harold Merskey of the National Hospital for Nervous Diseases, said:

> Of course, instruction in relaxation may have helped to diminish the physical causes of pain in the 'special case' group. But it is very likely that the psychological techniques which give the patients confidence, actually diminished the pain. In a way, this is a placebo response in which the friendly and comforting attitudes of the staff worked better than a placebo pill. It emphasizes the importance of a skilful psychological approach (or even just plain goodwill) in the nursing not only of psychiatric patients but also medical and surgical ones. . . . If the above is accepted – and there is much evidence to support it – it would seem that a humane and considerate approach will greatly ease the pain from which patients suffer without them needing to use excessive medication [*Nursing Times*, 12 August 1971].

It is upon these mental aspects of pain that I believe medical research should concentrate in the future. The secret of the yogas, who, in effect, 'switch off ' the pain of burning coals or spiky beds, deserves much more thorough investigation. Might not this power be acquired by ordinary people?

Personal control of pain may not be the only manoeuvre left in the battle. But it could certainly bring millions of people closer to victory.

Index